Edited by E.I. Hernández-Jiménez, E.M. Rakhanskaya

COMPREHENSIVE COSMETIC SKINCARE
IN COSMETIC DERMATOLOGY & SKINCARE PRACTICE

Cosmetics & Medicine
Publishing

Author/Editor:
Elena I. Hernández-Jiménez, *Ph.D.*

Editor:
Ekaterina M. Rakhanskaya, *M.D.* Neurologist, radiation safety specialist

Author:
Vera I. Albanova, *M.D., Ph.D., Prof.* Dermatologist

COMPREHENSIVE COSMETIC SKINCARE
IN COSMETIC DERMATOLOGY AND SKINCARE PRACTICE

Comprehensive skincare with the help of cosmetic products is the key to maintaining health and youthfulness. Even the most unproblematic skin needs care with properly selected cosmetic products that preserve the skin's own resources and help resist external influences that accelerate aging. Moreover, any popular injection or physical treatment can give maximum effect only if the patient consistently follows a professional and home-based skincare regimen. This is the responsibility of the skincare practitioner, who must be able to not only perform the cosmetic procedure but also help select and explain to the patient the importance of using suitable products for their skin type.

This book is dedicated to a detailed review and justification of the importance of all stages of cosmetic care for different skin types — preparation with cleansers and exfoliants, intensive action aimed both at stimulating metabolic processes in the skin and solving various aesthetic problems (e.g., rejuvenation, whitening), and completion of procedures with active cosmetic agents, thereby consolidating the results and increasing the renewed skin's protective potential. We explain in detail how classic and modern products work and why they can be used in some cases and are undesirable in others. We further discuss the most common questions that arise from skincare practitioners and their patients. In addition, separate sections of the book are devoted to skincare for the eyelids, lips, and hands.

The book is useful to all professionals working with skin — long-time specialists and novice skincare practitioners, dermatologists, and consultants in selling skincare products, as well as students. In addition, it is of interest to all people who want to have healthy and youthful skin — the publication will expand their understanding of what a beautician does, and why it is so important to provide the necessary care for the skin, and, of course, what exactly it should be.

ISBN 978-1-970196-18-4 (paperback)
ISBN 978-1-970196-12-2 (eBook – Adobe PDF)
ISBN 978-1-970196-17-7 (eBook – ePUB)

© Cosmetics & Medicine Publishing LLC, 2024
© Cover photo: Roman Samborskyi / Shutterstock

FirstEditing

English version is edited and certified by the FirstEditing.Com, Inc. (USA).

Author/Editor

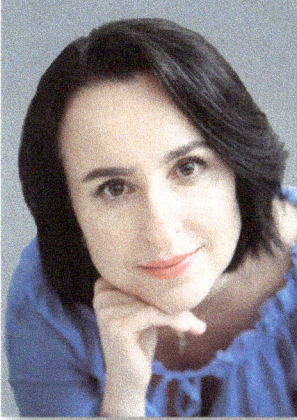

Elena I. Hernández-Jiménez, *Ph.D.*

Biophysicist, scientific journalist

Editor-in-chief of Cosmetics and Medicine Publishing

Chairperson of the Executive Board of the International Society of Applied Corneotherapy (I.A.C.)

Author and co-author of numerous publications in professional magazines, co-author and editor of the book series *Fundamentals of Cosmetic Dermatology & Skincare*, *Cosmetic Dermatology & Skincare Practice*, *Cosmetic Chemistry for Dermatology & Skincare Specialists* and others

Speaker at international conferences, author of training seminars and webinars for professionals in the field of skincare

Professional interests: biology and physiology of the skin, skin permeability, cosmetic chemistry, anti-age medicine, physiotherapy in dermatology and aesthetic medicine, skin analysis and imaging

Table of Contents

PART III
SPECIAL SKINCARE PRODUCTS AND TREATMENTS

Abbreviations

AHA — alpha-hydroxy acid
CGRP — calcitonin gene-related peptide
CRABP — cellular retinoic acid-binding protein
CRBP — cellular retinol-binding protein
DNA — deoxyribonucleic acid
DOPA — dioxyphenylalanine
EDTA — ethylenediaminetetetraacetic acid
FDA — Food and Drug Administration
FFA — free fatty acids
IL — interleukin
INCI — International Nomenclature of Cosmetic Ingredients
LHA — lipohydroxy acid
MMP — matrix metalloproteinases
MSH — melanocyte-stimulating hormone
NADP — nicotinamide adenine dinucleotide phosphate
NMF — natural moisturizing factor
PABA — para-aminobenzoic acid
pH — hydrogen index, a measure of the acidity of aqueous solutions
PHA — polyhydroxy acid
PM — suspended solids
RA — retinoic acid
RAR — retinoic acid receptor
RNA — ribonucleic acid
ROSs — reactive oxygen species
RXR — retinoid X receptor
SPF — sun protection factor
TCA — trichloracetic acid
TEWL — transepidermal water loss
UV — ultraviolet

Introduction

Even young and healthy skin needs care. Properly chosen cosmetic products can preserve the skin's resources and help resist external aging factors. Moreover, the effects of injection or physical treatments so popular nowadays would be enhanced if the client follows routine skincare. This book gives a detailed examination of the stages of comprehensive cosmetic skincare.

Although cosmetic procedures vary depending on the objectives and products used, we can distinguish four steps that are in one form or another included in all cosmetic care programs:

1. Preparation
2. Treatment
3. Restoration
4. Protection

At the **preparatory stage**, the skin is cleaned of makeup, dirt, and excess sebum, irregularities of the *stratum corneum* are removed, and the skin is prepared for applying subsequent products.

At the **treatment stage**, particular aesthetic problems are solved with the help of specific active formulations.

At the **recovery stage**, if necessary, the skincare practitioner removes residues of cosmetic products used at the previous stage, soothes the skin, and applies topical agents to help regenerate it.

Finally, in the **protective stage**, a protective cream containing ultraviolet (UV) filters (to reduce the UV load on the skin), antioxidants (to prevent severe inflammation), and occlusive components (this is especially important after procedures in which there is a temporary weakening of the barrier function) are applied to the skin.

But before delving into the stages of skincare, it is essential to dwell on the topic of skin classification issues because skin type largely determines the choice of specific products.

Part I

Skin types

Although skin structure is the same for all human beings, there is a difference in the realization of skin functions. Some have active sebaceous glands, some do not, some have heavily pigmented skin, some have poorly pigmented skin, some have sensitive skin, and some easily tolerate various factors. It turns out that, we need to create different cosmetic products to provide skincare that meets the needs of specific people.

Back in the early 1900s, entrepreneur and cosmetic formulator Helena Rubinstein proposed the first classification of skin types, which she imagined would describe the most common variants in people's skin and help to select the most appropriate skincare for them. According to her classification, all skin types can be divided into normal, oily, and dry. However, the more scientists learned about skin structure, the more they realized that this classification not only does not reflect all the options but is simply incorrect to use it to select care programs because, for example, dry skin can also be oily.

1.1. Classification according to sebum production and *stratum corneum*'s water content

The fact is that oily skin is an indicator of the intensity of the sebaceous glands, and dry skin is an indicator of the state of the barrier structures of the *stratum corneum*. In hypersecretion, sebum can "dilute" the lipid barrier, disturbing the ratio of physiological lipids in it, which increases skin permeability for chemicals, including water.

Thus, it is correct to distinguish two classifications.

According to **the level of sebum production:**
- Low-sebum skin
- Skin with a normal amount of sebum
- Oily skin (sebum overproduction)

In terms of **water content in the *stratum corneum*:**
- Dry skin (insufficient moisture)
- Skin with normal moisture level
- Hypermoisturized skin

There is also the **"dehydrated skin"** condition, which differs from **"dry skin."** Dry skin has compromised barrier properties at the *stratum corneum* level. In contrast, dehydrated skin has a water deficiency under the *stratum corneum* due to changes in the extracellular matrix of the dermis. At the same time, dry skin can have normal turgor, and dehydrated skin can have good barrier properties.

There are conditions when the skin has symptoms of dryness and dehydration. Such a combination can be observed, for example, in photodamaged skin because of the negative impact of UV rays on different skin layers and structures. In any case, the purpose of applying the cosmetic product is the normalization of the water content of the skin tissue. Still, methods of normalization of water balance and hydration differ dramatically, depending on the level of exposure and the nature of structural changes that have led to a water deficit. Cosmetics can help in the case of dry skin. However, in the case of dehydration, although strengthening the barrier function somewhat increases the moisture content of the skin as a whole, injectable procedures like mesotherapy and biorevitalization are more relevant.

Signs of oily skin:
- Greasy shine
- Enlarged pores
- Hyperkeratosis
- Good turgor
- Increased sensitivity and irritability
- Inflammation (for acne and seborrheic dermatitis)

Signs of dry skin:

- Visible scaling
- Roughness
- Feeling of tightness
- Superficial wrinkles
- Dullness
- Increased sensitivity and irritability (sometimes)

It is important to remember that these parameters are labile. **Skin dryness, like sebaceous gland activity, can change under the influence of both external and internal factors.**

1.2. Classification according to the tendency for irritation

Another variable parameter is skin sensitivity. In 2017, the International Forum for the Study of Itch (IFSI) defined sensitive skin as **a syndrome associated with unpleasant sensations (tingling, burning, pain, heat, and itching) in response to stimuli that should not provoke such sensations in highly-tolerant skin** (Misery L. et al., 2017). Although this definition is not yet standardized, it is accepted by many specialists worldwide because it most clearly reflects the essence of the "sensitive skin" phenomenon. According to this definition, skin is divided into **non-sensitive (resistant, highly-tolerant)** and **sensitive**. Sensitive skin is usually classified based on the main pathogenetic mechanisms that contribute to the development of sensitivity. For example, Japanese dermatologists suggested distinguishing the following three main types of sensitive skin (Yokota T. et al., 2003):

- **Unprotected skin** has a reduced barrier function. This type is characterized by increased transepidermal water loss (TEWL) and pathological desquamation.
- **Inflamed skin** has a tendency to inflammatory changes without a pronounced loss of barrier function of the epidermis.
- **Neurosensitive skin** has no inflammatory changes, the barrier function is normal, and all the problems come from within the body.

1.3. Classification according to melanin level and the ability to produce pigment

Skin is characterized by natural pigmentation, which is the genetically determined amount of melanin synthesized by melanocytes. However, the skin color itself can change with tanning. This pigmentation is called **acquired pigmentation**.

The best-known classification of pigmentation is the **Fitzpatrick scale of skin phototypes**. (Note that skin types and phototypes are often confused, even though they are distinct characteristics.) This classification was developed by the American dermatologist Thomas Fitzpatrick in 1975 and was subsequently modified slightly. It is based on the skin's response to UV radiation, that is the skin's ability to tan. It also reflects well the distribution of skin colors in general (**Fig. I-1-1**).

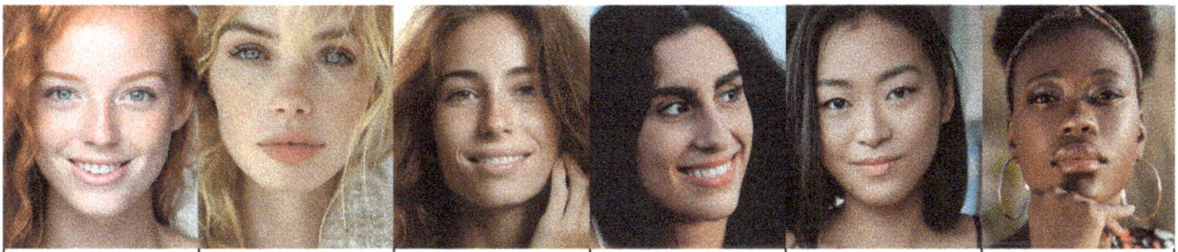

I Celtic	II Light-skinned Caucasian	III Dark-skinned Caucasian	V Mediter-ranean/ Asian	V Indone-sian/ Hindu	VI African
never tans, always burns	sometimes tans, often burns	always tans, sometimes burns	quickly tans, rarely burns	never tans, never burns	never tans, rarely burns
SPF 50	SPF 30–50	SPF 15–30	SPF 6–15	SPF 15	SPF 15
to prevent photodamage and photoaging				to prevent photoaging	

Figure I-1-1. Thomas Fitzpatrick's skin phototypes and sun protection product recommendations (Image by Freepik)

I.   Celtic — skin never tans, always burns (very light skin, blond or red hair, blue or green eyes, freckles)
II. Light-skinned Caucasian — sometimes manages to tan, but more often, skin burns (light skin, blond or brown hair, blue, green, or gray eyes)
III. Dark-skinned Caucasian — skin tans but sometimes burns (medium shade of skin from light to swarthy, dark brown or brown hair, usually brown eyes)
IV. Mediterranean/Asian — skin tans quickly, rarely burns (light brown skin, dark brown or brown hair, usually brown eyes)
V.   Indonesian/Hindu — skin never burns (very dark skin, black hair, black eyes)
VI. African — skin never burns (dark skin, black hair, black eyes)

Phototypes I and II are considered **melanocompromised** (no protection), while phototypes III and IV are **melanocompetent** (acquired protection), and phototypes V and VI are **melanoprotective** (innate protection).

Knowing your phototype lets you predict safe tanning time and choose the right sunscreen.

Fitzpatrick's classification is simple and accessible, making it easy to work with for patients. However, it does not consider the diversity of skin color and, important for skincare, the active mixing of races. The problem is that the descendants of light-skinned and dark-skinned people may have lighter natural pigmentation than their dark-skinned ancestors but respond to UV light just as intensely. Yet, they may, for example, be more prone to develop pigmentary defects (e.g., post-inflammatory hyperpigmentation, sun damage) than would be expected under Fitzpatrick's classification. One of the options for predicting such phenomena is the **Lancer ethnicity scale**, introduced in 1998 by Dr. Harold A. Lancer (Lancer H.A., 1998). This scale allows the phototype to be determined, taking into account heredity. The phototypes (according to Fitzpatrick) of two grandparents are summed and divided by four. This refinement helps to anticipate some of the side-effects of aggressive cosmetic procedures.

1.4. Classification according to the wrinkle appearance

Another parameter by which skin is classified is the presence of wrinkles. Accordingly, skin is divided into wrinkled and smooth. The wrinkles are divided into:

- Superficial fine lines
- Expression lines (due to facial muscles movement)
- Static wrinkles (persisting even at rest)
- Folds
- Furrows

The appearance of wrinkles mainly indicates changes in the dermal layer of the skin. Although it is not easy to influence its condition with cosmetic products, even superficial agents can slow the aging process, such as sunscreens that prevent photoaging, products that strengthen the barrier function, and anti-inflammatory and antioxidant components that inhibit inflammation-induced aging.

1.5. Baumann's four-criteria classification

Another well-known classification, the skin classification proposed by Leslie Baumann in 2004, should be mentioned separately. Baumann suggested grading the skin according to the following four criteria:

- Dry (**D**) or oily (**O**)
- Sensitive (**S**) or resistant (**R**)
- Pigmented (**P**) or unpigmented (**N**)
- Tight (**T**) or wrinkled (**W**)

The following 16 combinations of skin types are possible (**Table I-1-1**):
1. DRNT: dry, resistant, unpigmented, smooth
2. DRNW: dry, resistant, unpigmented, wrinkle-prone
3. DRPT: dry, resistant, pigmented, smooth
4. DRPW: dry, resistant, pigmented, wrinkle-prone
5. DSNT: dry, sensitive, unpigmented, smooth
6. DSNW: dry, sensitive, unpigmented, wrinkle-prone
7. DSPT: dry, sensitive, pigmented, smooth

8. DSPW: dry, sensitive, pigmented, wrinkle-prone
9. ORNT: oily, resistant, unpigmented, smooth
10. ORNW: oily, resistant, unpigmented, wrinkle-prone
11. ORPT: oily, resistant, pigmented, smooth
12. ORPW: oily, resistant, pigmented, wrinkle-prone
13. OSNT: oily, sensitive, unpigmented, smooth
14. OSNW: oily, sensitive, unpigmented, wrinkle-prone
15. OSPT: oily, sensitive, pigmented, smooth
16. OSPW: oily, sensitive, pigmented, wrinkle-prone

Table I-1-1. Baumann Skin Types

	OILY		DRY		
	Pigmented	Unpigmented	Pigmented	Unpigmented	
Sensitive	OSPW	OSNW	DSPW	DSNW	Wrinkled
Sensitive	OSPT	OSNT	DSPT	DSNT	Smooth
Resistant	ORPW	ORNW	DRPW	DRNW	Wrinkled
Resistant	ORPT	ORNT	DRPT	DRNT	Smooth

This classification is one of the most popular, based on which protocols have been created to select adequate and effective care. However, despite the advantages of such a comprehensive approach, it also initially divides skin into dry and oily, which does not always reflect the problem that needs to be addressed. Even if this classification treats truly dry skin (i.e., skin with a damaged skin barrier) as dry sensitive skin, this is not always the case either. Yes, in most cases, dry skin is accompanied by hypersensitivity, but sensitive skin is not always dry. Other causes play a role in hypersensitivity, and you can read more about them in our *Sensitive Skin in Cosmetic Dermatology & Skincare Practice* book.

Moreover, most mass-market products are still, unfortunately, guided by the classical skin classification, which does not consider all

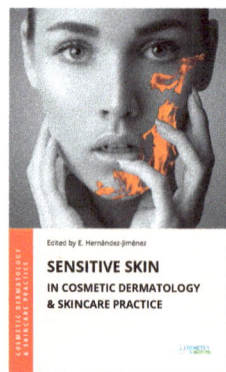

important features of skin physiology. That is why we have given a detailed description of the parameters, the evaluation of which makes it possible to choose the optimal skincare for a specific person. In addition, such an assessment makes it possible to record and dynamically evaluate the peculiarities of skin conditions. Most importantly, this approach allows us to see the efficiency of the chosen care.

It is essential to be aware that the skin type can change due to cosmetic care, dermatological treatment, or medication. If the correct program leads to the "normalization" of the skin type, the wrong care can aggravate problems and even cause the development of pathology.

Part II

Pre-treatment skin preparation

Cleansing the skin is one of the most important steps in a skincare routine. For many years it was believed that healthy skin means clean skin, so washing your skin almost "until it squeaks" was suggested. But this is the wrong strategy. Dissolution of the protective hydrolipidic layer of the skin and damage to the *stratum corneum* by detergents with aggressive surfactants contained in products for cleansing can lead to a violation of its barrier function, facilitate access to allergens and irritants, disrupt the normal process of epidermal regeneration, and make the skin defenseless against pathogenic microorganisms. Moreover, surfactants are also detrimental to the "healthy" microbiome — those microorganisms that permanently reside on our skin, forming synergistic relationships with it. In exchange for residence and nutrition, they protect against pathogenic microbes, strengthen the skin barrier, and help resist the negative impact of environmental factors.

Meanwhile, we cannot agree with some authors who advise not to wash at all, but to scrub dirt from the body with special spatulas, to anoint it with incense, and pour deodorants. A clean, well-groomed body is an indispensable feature of the appearance of a civilized person.

It should not be forgotten that women often have makeup on their faces, which still needs to be thoroughly washed off occasionally. Moreover, the skin of those living in megacities is exposed to large amounts of substances, such as air pollutants, which dissolve in lipids and cannot be washed away with water only. Their presence is not only undesirable, but is also dangerous for the skin because they provoke inflammatory reactions and oxidative stress. Finally, skin cleansing is especially important before any cosmetic procedures.

Chapter 1
The *stratum corneum* as the main skin barrier

The skin consists of three layers: epidermis, dermis, and hypodermis. The epidermis, in turn, consists of cell layers with different structures and functions. From a practical point of view, the outermost layer of the epidermis, the *stratum corneum*, is especially important because it gives skincare practitioners many problems.

The *stratum corneum* consists of flat corneocytes filled with keratin and surrounded by a protein-lipid envelope (cornified envelope). Cornified envelopes of neighboring cells are connected both by protein

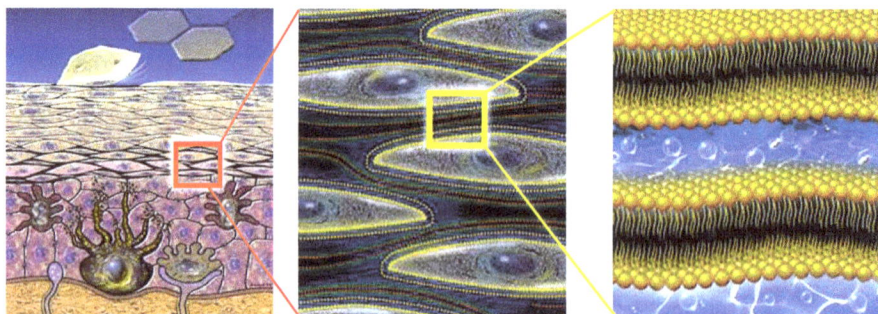

Keratinocyte reproduction occurs in the epidermis's lowest (basal and subbasal) layers. The newly formed cells move upwards, maturing and turning into horny scales (corneocytes).

The *stratum corneum* consists of densely packed corneocytes, between which there are lipid layers.

The lipid barrier of the *stratum corneum*, located between corneocytes, is the main skin permeability barrier. Its lipids (ceramides, fatty acids, cholesterol) and the water layers form a lamellar liquid crystalline system.

Figure II-1-1. The *stratum corneum*: a "brickwork" model (adapted from Skincare Forum Online, www.scf-online.com)

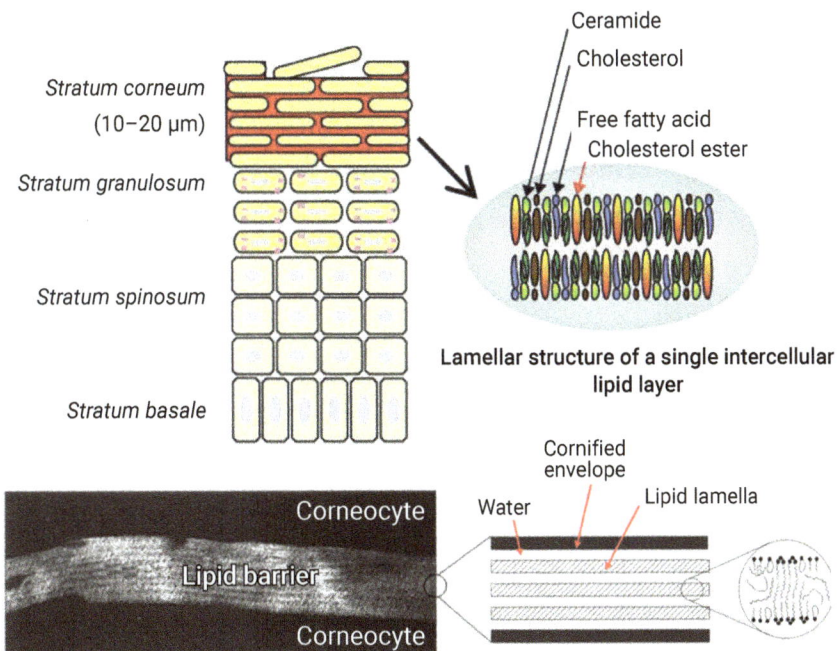

Figure II-1-2. Structure and composition of the lipid barrier

bridges (desmosomes) and fatty acid threads that "pierce" intercellular lipid layers of the *stratum corneum* (**Fig. II-1-1**).

Between the corneocytes are multilayered lipid layers organized into a "lipid barrier" structure. The lipid composition of the barrier is unique — nowhere else in the body is such a structure observed (**Fig. II-1-2**).

The barrier's main lipids are ceramides — accounting for almost 50% of the total volume. A high content of cholesterol and its esters — up to 18% (declining to only a few percent in living cells' membranes) — is characteristic of the barrier and unacceptable for membranes of living cells. Cholesterol is a viscosity regulator, and when its concentration deviates from the norm, lipid layers' fluidity changes dramatically, affecting their functionality. Finally, the third component of the lipid barrier are free fatty acids (accounting for 11–15%). They also influence the fluidity of lipid structures, but in addition, they perform other functions. For example, some fatty acids have bactericidal properties, and others are involved in additional stabilization of the lipid barrier, "sewing" neighboring layers with each other and with horn envelopes.

The *stratum corneum* protects our body from dehydration and penetration of foreign substances and microorganisms, but it also prevents the penetration of active ingredients of skincare products into the skin. And yet the *stratum corneum*, although reliable, is not an absolute protection against dehydration and foreign substances. Today we know that lipid layers are heterogeneous: there are areas in which lipids are densely packed, rendering them practically impermeable to water and water-soluble substances, and areas characterized by more liquid, free lipid packing, which have higher permeability. Depending on the composition of *stratum corneum*'s lipids, the ratio of "dense" and "liquid" areas changes, affecting the barrier's permeability and water-holding properties.

The corneocytes are flexible and malleable due to water. Compared to living cells with 80–90% water content, there is little water in corneocytes — about 10% of the scale's weight. Some of the water is inside corneocytes, being bound to keratin by electrostatic forces. Another part, bound to molecules of natural moisturizing factor (NMF) — a group of low-molecular-weight hygroscopic substances present only in the skin's *stratum corneum* — forms a hydrated shell around the corneocytes.

As the corneocytes wear away from the skin (special enzymes take part in this process), the top skin layer is constantly renewed. Because the uppermost layers of the *stratum corneum* are constantly exposed to external factors (including hot water and soap), the lipid layer is no longer as pronounced there. Instead, the space between the partially exfoliated *stratum corneum* is filled with sebum, makeup particles, and other types of dirt.

In addition, as we age, corneocytes exfoliate less effectively, and the *stratum corneum* becomes uneven — in some areas, it is thinner, while in others, it is thickened and has keratotic plaques. When oily skin exfoliates unevenly, corneocytes can form chaotic deposits stuck together by sebum and cream.

If cosmetic substances are applied to unprepared skin, the active ingredients linger within the *stratum corneum* instead of penetrating it. This circumstance becomes especially important in chemical peeling when the impact is made simultaneously on a large area. Penetration uniformity of peeling agents is one of the most important conditions for the success of a peeling procedure.

Thus, from an aesthetic point of view, skin cleansing is extremely important for daily preventive care and the expected future cosmetic manipulations.

Skin preparation for the procedure consists of the following steps:

1. **Cleansing** to remove makeup, sebum, and impurities from the skin
2. **Exfoliation** to even out the *stratum corneum* (enzymatic peeling, light superficial peeling with fruit acids, hydro-peel by strong stream of water solution, mechanical peeling by scrubs)
3. **Moisturizing** to increase the permeability of the *stratum corneum*

Let us dwell in more detail on the cosmetic products used at these steps.

Chapter 2
Skin cleansing and cleansers

Simply washing with water is not enough to effectively cleanse the skin — it removes up to 65% of sebum and impurities deposited on the skin surface, but it is not possible to completely clean the skin (including decorative cosmetics, which contain a lot of hydrophobic compounds) in this way. For this purpose, special cleansers containing emulsifiers and fat solvents are used.

2.1. Skin cleansers

2.1.1. Soap

Soap was the first hygiene product designed to cleanse the skin and hair. Soap, the main component of which is surfactants, in combination with water, is used either as a cosmetic product — for cleaning and skincare (toilet soap) or as a household detergent for cleaning various surfaces (laundry soap).

Principle of cleansing action

The essence of soap action is as follows. Surfactants of the soap solution penetrate hydrophobic deposits on the skin surface (which are a mixture of sebum, dust, and cosmetics) embedded into them, "crush" them into smaller particles, and envelop them, preventing re-deposition. Insoluble hydrophobic particles become suspended (their suspension in water is formed), after which they are easily washed away with water.

Soap chemistry

Many people today use the term "soap" to refer to a cosmetic cleanser without regard to its chemical nature. However, from a chemical point of view, this is not exactly true. Soaps (chunky and liquid) are divided into three basic types.

- **Natural soap** is usually a solid product which is a mixture of water-soluble salts of higher fatty acids (usually sodium, less often potassium and ammonium salts of acids such as stearic, palmitic, myristic, lauric, and oleic) and glycerol. Soap production is based on the reaction of saponification — hydrolysis of fatty acid esters with alkalis, which results in the formation of alkali metal salts and alcohols. Animal fat and vegetable oil, fat substitutes (synthetic fatty acids, rosin, naphthenic acids, tallow oil) can be used as raw materials to produce the main component of soap. Modern soaps are usually a mixture of fatty acids from tall and vegetable oils in the ratio of 4:1. Increasing the tall fraction causes an oily film to remain on the skin after washing (such soap is called superfatted soap). Superfatted soap may also contain lanolin and paraffin. Transparent soap is made by increasing the glycerin content and adding sucrose. The pH of natural soap is always alkaline and ranges from 9 to 11 (Boonchai W., Iamtharachai P., 2010).
- **Combination soap (combar)** consists of alkaline soap with other surfactants as additives; it has a pH of 9–10.
- **Synthetic soap (syndet)** is made from synthetic detergent. It can look like a natural soap, i.e., it can be in the form of a traditional solid bar (molded soap does not contain water), or it can be liquid. It consists of synthetic surfactants (often sodium lauryl isethionate) and fillers. It can also contain natural soap, but not more than 10%. The pH of such a product can be adjusted to the necessary level of 5.5–7.0 (citric or lactic acid is usually used for this purpose).

The most common surfactants of **solid soaps**:
- Sodium cocoate
- Sodium thaloate
- Sodium palmitate
- Sodium stearate
- Sodium cocoyl thionate
- Sodium isethionate
- Sodium dodecyl benzenesulfonate
- Sodium cocoglyceryl ether sulfonate
- Triethanolamine stearate

Surfactants of **liquid soap**:

- Diethanolamine (DEA) lauramide
- Sodium laureth sulfate
- Socamidopropyl betaine
- Sodium cocoilsethionate
- Sodium laureth sulfosuccinate

Both natural and synthetic soaps may include additives that increase the detergent capacity of the product and improve the dermatological characteristics (refatting agents, moisturizers) and appearance (dyes, fragrances). As for antiseptic additives like triclosan and triclocarban that act against skin microflora, their inclusion is currently considered inexpedient from a biological point of view:

1. They effectively destroy cells of microorganisms in a non-specific way (they break the integrity of their outer membrane).
2. During short-term contact with the skin, antibacterial additives hardly have time to realize their capabilities.

Antiseptics such as benzoyl peroxide and sulfur can be found in preparations for cleansing oily skin and skin with acne manifestations.

Dermatological aspects

The high alkalinity of natural soaps is a big disadvantage regarding the impact on the skin barrier. After washing with an alkaline solution, the pH on the skin's surface rises, and it takes an average of two hours for the skin to recover to its physiological "acidic" level.

In addition, salt ions in natural soaps can "wash out" the NMF molecules from the *stratum corneum*, and fatty acids can clog pores (especially if the skin is prone to forming comedones). Therefore, it is advisable to reduce the contact time of the soap solution with the skin and wash it off as soon as possible with plenty of water. If you cannot remove all the dirt in one go, it is better to soap the skin again rather than increase the time the soap solution is left on the skin.

Frequent use of natural soaps can also be detrimental to the skin — if the skin is exposed to soap before it has had time to regain its barrier structures, irritation and dryness can occur. There is an especially high risk of adverse reactions in the skin with a weakened barrier (e.g., due to skin diseases such as dermatitis and psoriasis) and hypersensitivity. In these cases, abandoning natural soaps and using their synthetic analogues (syndets), emulsions, or water-based cleansers is necessary.

The ability to adjust the pH of the finished product is a huge advantage of syndets over natural soaps and allows them to be used for damaged and/or sensitive skin. In addition, the surfactants of modern syndets act on the skin more gently than the surfactants of natural soaps.

In turn, additives in soaps (natural or synthetic) can cause unwanted reactions in the skin. Therefore, for cleaning delicate, sensitive and/or damaged skin, products with very few additives (at least without dyes and fragrances) are preferable.

Distribution

In recent years, using synthetic soaps (solid or liquid) for personal hygiene has become very popular. Natural soap is gradually moving from mass consumption into the niche sector — it is used by natural cosmetics manufacturers and author's products (the so-called "handmade soap").

The use of natural soap as a household cleaner is also decreasing worldwide, with consumers choosing detergents, dishwashers, and other products for cleaning a wide variety of surfaces.

2.1.2. Oil-free cleansers

This category includes fatty substances-free cleansers, e.g., water gels and cleansing solutions (tonics). They contain water, glycerin, cetyl alcohol, sterol alcohol, sodium lauryl sulfate, and (sometimes) propylene glycol.

The product is applied to dry or damp skin with the fingertips (or with a washcloth/sponge in the case of shower gel), after which the foam is whipped up and rinsed off with water. The foam dissolves and emulsifies grease and dirt on the skin's surface.

It is a gentle cleanser especially recommended for people with photodamaged skin. However, propylene glycol can lead to a feeling of tightness, so such products are not recommended for very dry skin. In addition, sodium lauryl sulfate, which provides foam formation, is one of the surfactants with increased irritant potential and is not recommended for skin with a severely damaged barrier.

2.1.3. Cleansing emulsions

Emulsion-based products such as cold cream (thick emulsion) and milk (liquid emulsion) can be used for cleansing the face and body. Like any emulsion, they contain three main substances: water, oils, and emulsifiers.

Although emulsifiers are chemically surfactants, they are used not to form foam but to prevent the water and oil phases from separating. Consequently, their concentration in emulsions is much lower than in soaps.

Cold cream

Cold cream is an emulsion of water-in-oil (w/o) type (water < 45%). It is called cold cream because of the cooling effect produced by water evaporation when this cream is applied to the skin.

The cooling effect depends not only on the water amount in the preparation but also on the type of fats and how the cream is prepared. In cold cream, the emulsifying agent is formed by a reaction between the alkaline sodium borate and the free fatty acids in white wax. Most cold creams emulsify large amounts of water by adding borax (sodium tetraborate decahydrate) or mucilaginous substances; for the same purpose, lanolin is added to the fat part of the preparation. Due to the abundance of water, cold cream spoils quickly. To prevent the rancidity, water is replaced by glycerin, but such a preparation is no longer essentially a cold cream. For example, a good, sufficiently stable cold cream can be obtained by mixing equal parts of lanolin, almond oil, and water (the amount of water can be further increased) and adding fragrant substances (rose oil). In modern preparations, mineral oil, petroleum jelly, and waxes (beeswax, vegetable, synthetic) can be found in the fat fraction of cold cream.

When applied to the skin, some fat components penetrate the intercellular spaces of the *stratum corneum*, and some remain on the surface, softening and moisturizing the skin due to the occlusion phenomenon (TEWL inhibition and water accumulation within the *stratum corneum*). At the same time, water contained in the preparation evaporates quickly, making the skin feel cool. Cold creams are very popular among patients with dry and irritated skin.

Cleansing milk

Cleansing milk is a light o/w emulsion. It is often used to remove makeup and cleanse delicate face areas, such as around the eyes and lips. To this end, it is applied directly to the skin and massaged gently with the fingertips, or it is first applied to a cotton pad and wiped over the skin. The treated area is rinsed with water or thoroughly wiped with a clean cotton pad dipped in water.

2.1.4. Hydrophilic oil

Hydrophilic oil comes from the Asian cosmetic market and is essentially a "do-it-yourself" emulsion. The product contains oils and emulsifiers, which are incorporated into the fatty impurities on the skin surface, "diluting" them, making them less dense, and crushing them into smaller particles. The hydrophilic "tails" of emulsifiers that can easily encounter water molecules remain "sticking out" on the surface of such lipid masses. Accordingly, when after oil application, a person begins to wash, rubbing water on the skin, these "tails" are "picked up" together with impurities and lipids dissolved in them, forming an emulsion during the washing. The well-balanced hydrophilic oil formulas rinse off perfectly, so there is no need to use other cleansers.

2.1.5. Micellar solution

The micellar solution is another popular type of skin cleanser. However, it does not contain the classic aggressive surfactants and is water-containing micelles composed of lipids. When applied to the skin, the micelle lipids also incorporate into the fatty plaques and crush them. Of course, micellar water can never be as effective as soap, which has a powerful cleansing effect due to the surfactants it contains. But such water is for sensitive skin — regular use does cleanse the skin, though not as well as products with active surfactants. **However, it is important to remember that micellar solution needs to be rinsed off just like other cleansers.**

The skin's barrier structures are located within the *stratum corneum* (the so-called **lipid barrier** composed of multi-layered lipid sheets between the *stratum corneum* scales) and on its surface (the **Marchionini mantle**, a mixture of sweat and sebaceous gland secretions, which covers the skin and has pH 4.5–5.5). Therefore, when cleansing the skin, it is necessary to take care not to cause severe damage to its barrier structures but rather to create optimal conditions for the qualitative restoration of its protective barrier.

The modern cosmetic industry offers many products for skin cleansing, differing in composition and principle of action. When choosing a skincare product, it is necessary to consider both the type of dirt and the condition of the skin — its barrier properties (the presence of damage, dryness), the intensity of sebum production, and sensitivity.

2.2. Factors determining the irritant potential of a cleanser

2.2.1. pH value

The main irritating factor of a cleanser formulation is the pH value. Thanks to the active advertising of skincare products with a pH of 5.5, many consumers believe this is the pH of a healthy skin surface. However, this is not entirely true.

First, what is pH? It is a convenient measure of acidity, calculated as the inverse decimal logarithm of the concentration of hydrogen ions (protons) in each solution. The higher the concentration of protons, the greater the acidity. But since the logarithm is inverse, the lower the pH value, the higher the acidity. Neutral solutions have a pH of 7.0. Anything below 7.0 is acidic, and anything above that is alkaline.

Human cells prefer a slightly alkaline environment — at pH 7.1–7.4. Living skin cells are no exception. The intercellular fluid, intracellular cytoplasm, and blood plasma have normal pH values in the slightly alkaline range. However, the skin's surface is covered by a layer of dead cells that protect it like a lizard is protected by its scales. Only here, in the *stratum corneum*, where there are no living cells, does the pH fall below neutral. The acidic pH on the skin's surface is created and maintained by the hydrolipid mantle that covers the skin. Its composition includes:

1. Substances that are secreted onto the skin surface as part of sebum and sweat. These are lactic and butyric acids from sweat, as well as cholesterol sulfate and free fatty acids from sebum, which are broken down to form acidic substances.
2. Metabolic products of NMF such as sodium pyroglutamate and urea.
3. Products of bacteria living on the skin. In particular, lactic acid bacteria secrete lactic acid.
4. Hydrogen ions generated during the operation of cellular ion pumps, such as the sodium pump.
5. Carbon dioxide, some of which escapes directly from the epidermis into the atmosphere and dissolves in the hydrolipid mantle to form carbon dioxide.

Based on this, we can assume that the pH can deviate from 5.5 since the activity of sweat and sebaceous glands and the composition of microorganisms varies on different parts of the body. And this is indeed the case. The commonly referenced value of 5.5 was determined for the armpit area, where the conditions vary considerably relative to other body parts due to highly active sweat glands. In fact, the skin on the back of the palm and the skin on the scalp have approximately similar pH values. However, pH is lower in other parts of the body, with the lowest values noted for the face, particularly the forehead (**Fig. II-2-1**) (Kleesz P. et al., 2012). Thus, when talking about the pH of the skin surface, it would be more correct to consider it as a range (i.e., 4.5–5.5).

In recent years, scientists' interest in the role of the skin's acid mantle (the so-called Marchionini mantle, named after the scientist who first described it) has increased significantly, and it has become clearer why it is so important for skin health (Surber C. et al., 2018).

Studies have shown that the pH gradient through the *stratum corneum* (at the surface, the pH value averages 4.5–5.5, as we have already mentioned, and at the border with the granular layer, it is already 7.0) regulates the keratinization and desquamation processes. The fact is that different enzymes work at different levels of the *stratum corneum*.

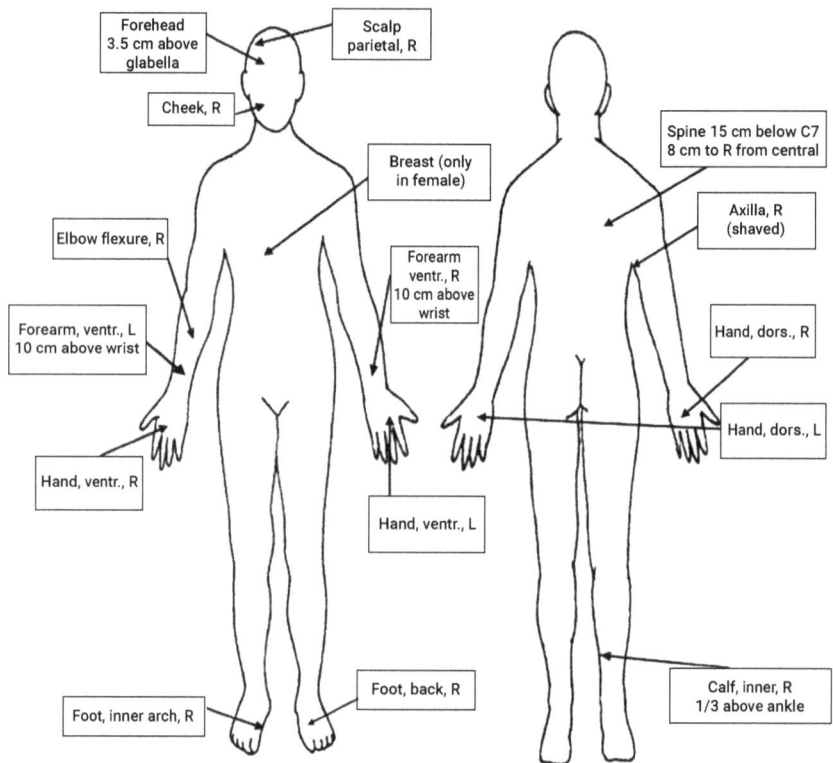

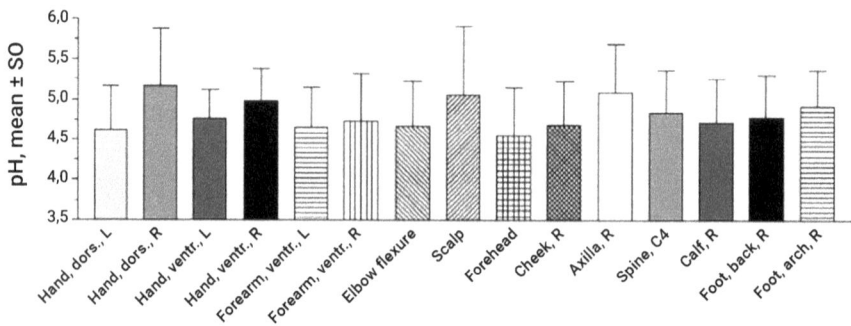

Figure II-2-1. Skin surface pH in different areas of the body (adapted from Kleesz P. et al., 2012)

At the surface, proteases are active, splitting corneodesmosomes (protein "bridges" that bind corneocytes to one another) so that the scales peel off in time. Intercellular lipid structures are formed in deeper layers, and other enzymes work in this area. The peculiarity of any enzyme is pH sensitivity — for each enzyme, there is a pH range within which the enzyme is most active. For example, for enzymes that regulate desquamation near the surface of the *stratum corneum*, the optimal pH is about 5.0. The optimum is shifted to the alkaline side for deeper enzymes and becomes about 6.0–7.0. Thus, **the pH gradient is a kind of "switch" that strictly controls the activity of enzymes in different areas of the *stratum corneum*.** If the physiological pH gradient is broken, there is a failure in the fine-tuned mechanisms of maturation and desquamation, resulting in a violation of the *stratum corneum* structure. This happens when the skin is exposed to acidic products (based on fruit acids) or when washing with alkaline soaps. The work of the enzyme structures is disturbed, which is expressed in the form of scaling and increasing skin dryness after some time. If you irrigate the skin with a neutral pH solution after the barrier has been destroyed, the barrier recovery slows down. Conversely, in an acidified environment, the barrier repairs faster.

The other role of the acid mantle is much better known: it regulates the microbial community living on our skin. A pH of 4.5–5.5 supports normal microflora. When the pH rises above normal values, the microbiological balance is disturbed, immediately affecting skin health. In particular, acne is characterized by a pH of about 6.0, which favors the excessive growth of *Cutibacterium acnes*. In atopic dermatitis, the surface pH of the skin is often elevated, and the microflora has a different composition than normal. An elevated pH creates a favorable environment for the development of purulent bacteria and fungi.

Experiments have shown that washing and applying skincare products have the most noticeable effect on skin surface pH. After washing with tap water, the skin takes an average of four hours to recover its pH. If soap is used when washing, this interval increases. When cosmetic products with a pH greater than 6.0 or less than 4.0 are used, the pH gradient in the *stratum corneum* is also shifted, sometimes on purpose. **Table II-2-1** presents the results of some studies on the changes in skin surface pH following a single cleansing treatment.

The appropriateness of affecting the skin by changing the pH gradient in the *stratum corneum* is determined in other stages of skincare treatment. This is not the task of cleansers, so their pH should not affect the intrinsic pH of the *stratum corneum*.

Table II-2-1. Changes in skin surface pH as a result of a single cleansing procedure (experimental data)

STUDY	CHANGES IN SKIN SURFACE pH AFTER A SINGLE CLEANSING TREATMENT
n = 40 (10 per means) Age: from 2 weeks to 16 months Gender: female/male Skin type: baby skin (Gfatter R. et al., 1997)	pH changes: • + 0.20 pH units (water) • + 0.29 pH units (cleanser) • + 0.45 pH units (alkaline soap) pH recovery time has not been calculated
n = 8 Age: 17–40 Gender: female Skin condition: healthy (Tamburic S., 1999)	pH changes: • + 0.5 pH units (product pH: 6.9–7.5) • + 2.0 pH units (product pH: 10.2–10.5) pH recovery: • pH has not been restored within 60 minutes (pH of the medium: 6.9–7.5) • pH remained elevated after 60 min (product pH: 10.2–10.5)
n = 48 Age: 17–59 Gender: female Skin condition: healthy (Gunathilake H.M. et al., 2007)	pH changes: • + 1.7 pH units (soap) • + 0.8 pH units (sindet) pH recovery: • pH restored within 60 min after washing (cleanser) • pH remained elevated after 60 min (soap)
n = 120 (20 per medium) Age: 20–25 Gender: female/male Skin condition: healthy (Moldovan M. et al., 2010)	pH changes: • + 2.1 to + 2.4 pH units (soap) • + 1.0 and + 1.3 pH units (sindet and combar) pH recovery: • pH remained elevated after 90 minutes (for every tested medium)
n = 63 Age: 40–65 Gender: female/male Skin condition: healthy (Aßmus U., et al., 2013)	pH changes: • + 1.07 pH units (water) • + 1.23 pH units (sindet: pH 7.0) • + 1.03 to + 1.17 pH units (sindet: pH 4.5)* pH recovery time has not been calculated

*The authors of the study note that despite the initial acidic pH of the syndet, its effect on skin surface pH is also determined by the surfactants included in it.

2.2.2. Surfactants

Even if the pH value corresponds to the physiological level, it is still impossible to consider any cleanser 100% safe and dermatologically mild simply because the main functional agents in most formulations are surfactants, which are necessary as without them, the product does not work.

The ability to dissolve (emulsify) fats makes surfactants a mandatory component of the vast majority of cleansers. But since both the membranes of living cells and the lipids of the epidermal barrier are also fats by their chemical composition, a sad conclusion can be drawn: **all products that cleanse the skin well can damage the epidermal barrier and cell membranes**.

Surfactants are compounds with **an amphiphilic structure**, i.e., their molecules have a polar part — a hydrophilic component (e.g., functional groups –OH, –COOH, –O–) and a non-polar (hydrocarbon) part — a hydrophobic (lipophilic) component. In an aqueous environment, the lipophilic part is embedded in the skin fat and pollution on the skin surface, while the hydrophilic part faces the water so that the insoluble particle surrounded on all sides detaches from the skin surface and passes into solution and is then washed off (**Fig. II-2-2**).

Surfactants differ in length, charge, and emulsifying power. The "strongest" surfactants are those contained in detergents with high foaming action. Even if the skin is characterized by increased sebum secretion, prolonged contact with surfactants should be avoided. Otherwise, the skin's barrier structures and acid mantle can be damaged.

Some surfactants decompose into ions in an aqueous solution: anionic surfactants carry a negative charge, cationic surfactants

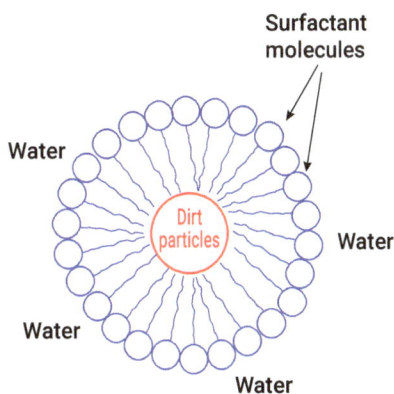

Figure II-2-2. Solubilizing effect of surfactants: contamination particle coated with surfactant molecules in an aqueous solution

Figure II-2-3. Schematic representation of (A) a phospholipid micelle in aqueous solution and (B) micellar solution

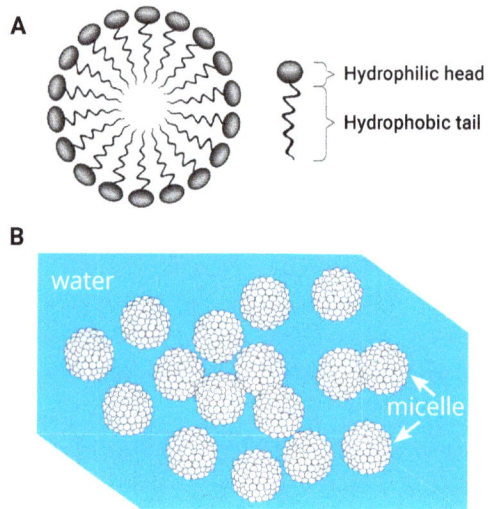

Micelles are particles in colloidal systems, consisting of a very small core insoluble in a given medium, surrounded by a stabilizing shell of adsorbed ions and solvent molecules. The average micelle diameter ranges from 1 to 100 nm. Micelles also include particles in solutions of surfactants called lyophilic colloids, e.g., micelles of lauryl sulfate in water.

carry a positive charge, and amphoteric surfactants carry both charges (zwitterions). Other surfactants dissolve in water without being ionized (these are the so-called non-ionic surfactants). Cationic surfactants are the most dangerous for the skin — they are hardly ever used in modern cosmetic products.

In emulsions, surfactants are located at the interface between the water and oil phases, forming a boundary layer. This layer prevents droplet coalescence and phase separation. In solution, surfactants can form micelles (Latin *mica* — particle) (**Fig. II-2-3**).

Anionic surfactants

Anionic surfactants are characterized by high foaming and cleansing power but can cause irritation. They are combined with mild surfactants and/or conditioning agents to reduce the irritating potential of the finished product. The mildest anionic surfactants are:

- Acyl phosphates
- Acyl sarcosinates
- Acyl taurates
- Isethionates
- Sulfoacetates

It is recommended to **avoid** the following anionic surfactants:

- Alkyl sulfates
- Lauryl sulfates (sodium lauryl sulfate)
- Ammonium lauryl sulfate
- Triethanolamine lauryl sulfate
- Olefinsulfates, fatty acid salts (soaps)
- Alkylarylsulfonates (the "toughest")

Amphoteric surfactants (zwitterions)

Amphoteric surfactants (zwitterions) are softer than anionic surfactants, but their pH can vary considerably. They are usually used as conditioning agents.

Non-ionic surfactants

Non-ionic surfactants are the mildest surfactants that tend to suppress foaming. They are included in products for children and for individuals with severely damaged skin. Among the most common soft surfactants (amphoteric and non-inogenic) are the following:

- Alkylated amino acids
- Alkylamines
- Cocamidopropyl betaine
- Sodium lauroamphoacetate
- Sodium cocoamphopropionate
- Cocoamino propionic acid
- Sodium lauraminopropionate
- Polyoxyethylated fatty alcohols
- Polyoxyethylated sorbitol esters
- Alkanolamides
- Poloxamers
- Alkylglycosides

Irritation potential of surfactants

Surfactants vary significantly in their irritant potential, which is mainly determined by their ability to bind to skin proteins and their penetration depth into the *stratum corneum*. Anionic (negatively charged) sulfate-based surfactants with short hydrophobic "tails" have the greatest irritating effect. These include sodium lauryl sulfate, which is a "standard irritant." As we have said, scientists usually use sodium lauryl sulfate in experiments to initiate skin irritation. However, the irritant effect severity of anionic and short-chain surfactants correlates with their concentration in the formulation and the presence of other ingredients, such as glycerol or betaine.

Since the irritating potential of a cleanser is determined by the composition of the surfactants, choosing these substances is particularly important when formulating a cleanser for sensitive skin with a weak or damaged barrier. This is not an easy task since most mild surfactants either do not form a good foam, give a sufficiently stable foam, or generally do not have the best cleansing capacity. One solution to this problem is to combine sulfate-based anionic surfactants (which can irritate the skin) with softer surfactants and betaine, which reduces the concentration and, therefore, the irritating potential of the basic surfactants while providing a good, stable foam. An esterified version of the anionic surfactants with a longer "tail" is also often used to make the product less damaging to the skin.

At the beginning of the 21st century, a group of very mild surfactants based on amino acids, particularly glutamic acid, appeared on the cosmetic market. They are beneficial because, along with good foaming properties, they do not damage the skin and even have moisturizing properties. Representatives of this category of surfactants are sodium cocoyl glutamate and sodium lauroyl oat amino acids.

Cleansing agents based on surfactants can work in the presence of water only. It is no exaggeration to say that **water is the main activator of a cleanser**.

The irritation potential of the cleanser is influenced by the presence of so-called **technical additives — dyes and fragrances**. The risk of irritation can be reduced by including moisturizing agents — in this case, glycerin is best (see below).

It is also important to know how well the detergent washes off the skin. Many problems are caused by substances that remain on the skin's surface, which then slowly migrate to the deeper layers. Only products that are easily removed by rinsing with water should be used for sensitive skin.

When formulating a product, remember that the softness of surfactants often depends on the other ingredients (**Table II-2-2**). For example, a successful combination of several surfactants can result in a softer product than if one surfactant is used. On the other hand, proteins, resins, and polymeric components can also reduce the irritant potential of the product.

Table II-2-2. Cleansing formulation components

SUBSTANCE	FUNCTION	PRODUCT
Water	• Dissolves and washes away dirt • Moisturizes and softens the skin • In skincare products, it forms an aqueous phase in which water-soluble substances present in the formulation are dissolved	Liquid soaps, cleansing gels, solutions, emulsions
Surfactants (anionic, amphoteric, non-ionic)	As a detergent: • crush hydrophobic deposits on the surface of the skin, resulting in a suspension of microparticles in the water, which is easy to rinse off	Natural and synthetic soaps
	As an emulsifier: • stabilize the emulsion, preventing its separation	Emulsions, scrubs
	As a foaming agent: • form a cleansing foam that emulsifies grease when combined with water	Natural and synthetic soaps; foams and self-foaming emulsions
Humectants (glycerin, polyquaternium-7, polyquaternium-10, chitosan)	Restore the necessary level of water in the *stratum corneum* and maintain its barrier properties	Emulsion-based products, oil-free water-based products, synthetic soaps

Continued on p. 42

SUBSTANCE	FUNCTION	PRODUCT
Conditioners (proteins, amphoteric surfactants)	Reduce the irritant potential of the product	Liquid detergents, emulsions, scrubs
Viscosity adjusters (polyols)	Regulate the viscosity of the finished product	Liquid detergents
Fillers	Prevent chunky soap from getting soaked	Solid soap
Preservatives	Prevent the growth of microorganisms in the product and its biological decomposition (spoilage)	Emulsion-based, oil-free, water-based products
Fragrances	Mask the smell of other compounds and give the product a pleasant aroma	In all cosmetic products
Dyes	Tint the product	In all cosmetic products
Antibacterial agents	Suppress the growth of micro-organisms	For cleansing products with claimed antibacterial properties: • for acne-prone skin (benzoyl peroxide) • for oily skin (sulfur) • antibacterial soap (triclosan, triclocarban)
Exfoliating agents (hydroxy acids, abrasives)	Help to soften and remove corneocyte buildup. Designed to care for skin with hyperkeratosis	• Glycolic acid and lactic acid — emulsion-based preparations, solutions (lotions) • Abrasives in scrubs

2.3. Additives in skin cleansers

2.3.1. Moistening agents

Many modern cleansers include substances that help temporarily "lock in" moisture on the skin's surface, preventing its rapid evaporation (and hence the feeling of tightness), and bind to corneocytes, keeping the *stratum corneum* soft and flexible and preventing it from cracking. Such additives are particularly important in industrial skin cleansers since they significantly reduce the discomfort caused by aggressive surfactants, solvents, and cleansers aimed for children, which often come in contact with already damaged and irritated skin. These products have limited use in professional cosmetic treatments, as they can leave a film on the skin that makes it difficult for the active ingredients to penetrate. On the contrary, they can reduce the risk of irritation in dry and sensitive skin.

The most common moisturizing ingredient in detergents is glycerin. We now know that glycerin plays an important role in transporting water through the protein channels of cell membranes, the so-called aquaporins, so its inclusion in cleansers is quite reasonable. Hydrating additives include mineral oil, moisturizing factor components (amino acids, minerals), aloe gel, proteins, fatty alcohols (stearyl alcohol), propylene glycol, waxes, silicones (dimethicone), and natural oils.

2.3.2. Calming agents

Since many negative reactions after washing are caused by signaling molecules released from keratinocytes, skin immunocytes, or nerve endings, using plant extracts with inflammation-blocking active ingredients can prevent or alleviate reactions such as itching, redness, and tingling. For this purpose, various additives are included in the formulation, which may include extracts of white willow, plantain, elderberry, algae, aloe, sea buckthorn, calendula, and other plants.

2.4. Choosing a cleanser

As we have discussed before, the paradigm of harsh cleansing, even for oily skin, is gradually becoming a thing of the past. Nowadays, cosmetic formulators and experts understand that it is important to maintain the skin barrier regardless of skin type. Therefore, using products with aggressive surfactants or alcohol that can damage it is no longer advised. Preference is given to gentle products.

The specific choice of cleanser should be based on the intensity of sebum production. If there is excessive sebum secretion, the choice should be a "soap-free" product (non-soap cleanser) that does not contain fatty acid salts (no more than 10% of these substances are allowed). For skin that does not produce enough sebum, a light emulsion — the so-called cosmetic milk, which contains emollients — is preferable. In all cases, without exception, the pH of the cleanser must be slightly acidic and should correspond to the physiological pH of the skin surface — not higher than 5.5.

- **The skin is normal or tends to be dry.** You can use cosmetic milk or a micellar solution for skin with normal or slightly reduced sebum levels. However, while cosmetic milk can be removed with sponges, **micellar solution must be rinsed from the skin**! Such mild cleansing base of emulsions can usually be enriched with soothing and relaxing extracts (calendula, rose, mallow) and softening components — apricot kernel oil and glycerin.
- **Dry skin.** For low-sebum dry skin, mild soap-free cleansers based on micellar solutions or light emulsions (cosmetic milk) are recommended, without traditional surfactants and alcohol, containing anti-inflammatory substances (e.g., plant extracts from chamomile, arnica, calendula, aloe). In this case, a creamy, low-foaming, soap-free cleanser may be the best choice, since it cleanses and moisturizes the skin.
- **Oily skin.** You should choose a dermatologically mild soap for skin with excessive sebum production, preferably syndet. It can be solid or liquid, but the main thing is that it has no fatty acid salts, and its solution in water has a pH not exceeding 5.5. But it should not be rubbed into the skin and left for a long time on

the face. If the dirt is not completely removed with one application, it is better to soap it a few times and rinse thoroughly with warm water. Products with salicylic acid can also be used for oily skin prone to scaling.

2.5. Skin exfoliation and exfoliating agents

After cleansing the skin, focus should shift to smoothing the *stratum corneum* and removing the top layer of corneocytes. For this purpose, various methods of skin exfoliation are used. The most popular are microdermabrasion and enzymatic peeling.

2.5.1. Scrubs

Microdermabrasion is a procedure aimed at evening the *stratum corneum* by applying abrasive particles. It can be carried out using a special microdermabrasion device or a scrub — a cosmetic product with abrasive particles. Scrub application to the skin is accompanied by light massaging movements, allowing the particles to seemingly roll over the skin's surface, "peeling off" the surface scales, which are already almost ready for desquamation. **Scrubs are not recommended for people with sensitive skin**.

Scrubs are **designed for**:
- Cleansing the face and body of surface impurities and accumulations of corneocyte masses
- Preparing the skin for the subsequent application of other cosmetic products
- Light massage and stimulation blood circulation
- Stimulation the epidermal renewal

Abrasive particles vary in hardness, size, and shape. If the particles are large, hard, and irregularly shaped, they can damage the skin and cause irritation. Too soft and fine particles, on the other hand, may not cleanse the skin well enough. The best scrubs are those with rounded abrasive particles (e.g., polyethylene granules or ground shells). The abrasive material can be made of:

- Crushed shells of seeds (e.g., apricots, almonds, grapes, peaches, walnuts)
- Solid waxes (e.g., jojoba wax granules, beeswax)
- Synthetic materials (e.g., polyethylene pellets, cellulose, nylon powder)
- Pumice stone (porous glassy volcanic rock)

Scrubs are divided into two groups according to their base: water- and oil-based scrubs. Water-based scrubs can be in the form of gel, paste, or milk. There is no fundamental difference between them. It is just a matter of personal preference. Due to the presence of the water phase, water-soluble biologically active additives, including proteolytic enzymes, bioflavonoids, and protein hydrolysates, can be included in the formulation. This makes it possible to combine skin cleansing with skin softening and moisturizing.

Oil-based scrubs contain salt or sugar crystals as abrasives. Mineral oil (a petroleum product), natural (vegetable), and synthetic oils (including silicone oils) can be used as a base. Natural oils in their pure form in the composition of scrubs are rare. First, they are easily oxidized (go rancid); second, applying and distributing them on the skin is more difficult. From this point of view, mineral oil or paraffin is preferred — these substances are biologically and chemically inert (and therefore do not cause allergies and dermatitis), odorless, and colorless, and are easily distributed on the skin.

To attract customers, oil-based scrubs sometimes contain essential oils. People with sensitive skin should avoid such products as, after cleansing and massage, the skin becomes more permeable, and the risk of irritation from essential oils increases.

Salt scrubs

Salt scrubs contain salts obtained from various natural sources (e.g., Himalayan salt, ocean salt, Dead Sea salt), but there are also products with ordinary table salt (sodium chloride). The main advantage of salt scrubs is a detoxifying effect (on the principle of exchange) and saturation of the skin with minerals (in the case of natural salts with a complex mineral composition). Products with sea salt not only cleanse the skin and provide it with the necessary minerals. The local increase in salt concentration within the *stratum corneum* "attracts" additional water, which tends to dilute the salt and reduce the osmotic force — as a result, the *stratum corneum* becomes moisturized. Salt scrubs stimulate circulation and metabolism and prepare the skin for anti-cellulite treatments. However, salt particles are hard, sharp-edged, and do not dissolve quickly, which produces a strong abrasive effect, so salt scrubs are only used in body treatments.

Sugar scrubs

Sugar scrubs are less popular and do not contain minerals. However, they have an important advantage — they are softer because the sugar particles do not have sharp edges and quickly dissolve in water. Sugar scrubs are recommended for facial skin and good moisturizing.

Usually, oil-salt and oil-sugar scrubs stratify because the heavy sugar or salt particles sink to the bottom. Therefore, they need to be stirred before application. Gel-forming additives such as powdered silicon and other substances are added to make the mixture of salt (sugar) and oil base look homogeneous.

More recently, polyglycols (propylene glycol, butylene glycol, polyethylene glycol) and high-molecular-weight silicone oils started to be used as a base for salt scrubs. All polyglycols are chemically inert, colorless (so they can be easily colored if required), and well dispersed on the skin. The interesting thing about polyglycols is that they heat up as they interact with water. Therefore, when washing the composition from the skin, a person feels a pleasant warmth. Silicone-based scrubs are also easily spread on the skin and leave a pleasant feeling after washing, thanks to the thin silicone film that remains on the surface — this film gives a silky feeling and a pleasant shine. Glycolic and silicone scrubs can be supplemented with emollients (to improve the sensation after scrub use), minerals, and other biologically active additives.

2.5.2. Enzymatic peeling

For people with sensitive skin and marked roughness of the *stratum corneum*, enzymatic exfoliation (syn.: enzymatic peeling) is indicated. Enzymatic peels do not have a chemical irritant effect like AHAs or a mechanical irritant effect like scrubs. Moreover, enzymatic peels fit perfectly into the concept of physiological skincare products because they mimic the skin's natural exfoliation mechanisms.

Several types of proteolytic enzymes capable of cleaving proteins are found in the *stratum corneum*, but two serine proteases — chymotrypsin-like and trypsin-like — play the leading role in the exfoliation process. One of the reasons for the delayed renewal of the *stratum corneum*, which is three to four days on average, is a decrease in the activity of proteolytic enzymes that break down the corneodesmosomes. As a result, conglomerates consisting of corneocyte masses, sebum, and impurities accumulate on the skin surface, making the skin look dull and acquire a grayish tint.

Unlike AHAs, which do not destroy anything directly, as they act indirectly by changing the pH gradient (see Part II, section 2.2, and Part III, section 1.5), proteolytic enzymes are based on destruction — they hydrolyze corneoodesmosomal proteins. Therefore, they can be classified as keratolytics (substances that denature the proteins of the *stratum corneum*), but with the caveat that their action is selective — they act exclusively on the proteins of the corneodesmosomes. This makes proteolytic enzymes fundamentally different from phenol, trichloracetic acid (TCA), and even salicylic acid, which non-selectively break intra- and intermolecular bonds of any proteins, causing their denaturation and destruction.

Enzymatic cleaners are the only category of skincare products in which enzymes are at least biologically appropriate. Proteolytic enzymes "work" on the skin's surface by loosening the adhesion of corneocytes by destroying the structural chemical bonds of corneodesmosomes and facilitating the exfoliation of corneocytes. Let us especially emphasize that such cosmetic formulations were initially created to keep the enzymes active rather than "push" them deep into the skin.

Most often, enzymatic peels include **proteolytic enzymes of plant origin**, such as papain, bromelain, and ficin. These enzymes belong to the cysteine proteases with the amino acid cysteine in their active center. In addition, the papain and bromelain fractions have some lipolytic activity.

Papain is a hydrolytic enzyme found in all parts of the melon tree (papaya) *Carica papaya* (except the roots), with the maximum amount found in immature fruits. Papain is interesting because it is the only cysteine protease with exopeptidase activity, i.e., it "bites off" a protein from the ends of the chain and can therefore break it down to its original amino acids. All other plant cysteine proteases used in skincare are endopeptidases, and the product of their activity are peptides of different sizes, not free amino acids. A papain molecule has a mass of 20.7 kDa, i.e., it is a relatively small protein in size, just like most other cysteine proteases. But even such a "modest" size significantly limits its penetration into the skin. Interestingly, papain needs activators to make it work. In the skin, such activators are cysteine and glutathione; in cosmetic products, they can be sodium thiosulfate, thioglycolic acid, and metal chelators (for example, EDTA).

Papain can hydrolyze almost all peptide bonds except those formed by proline residues. Nonetheless, it pays special "attention" to bonds formed by glycine, hydrophobic amino acids leucine, isoleucine, aromatic amino acids tyrosine, phenylalanine, and aspartic, glutamic, and cysteic acids. These amino acids are rich in the class of human keratin proteins and form the *stratum corneum* of the epidermis, hair, and nails (Brocklehurst K., Philpott M.P., 2013).

Besides papain, papaya's latex (milky juice) contains other cysteine proteases: **chymopapains A** and **B**, **peptidases A** and **B**, and **caricain**. These enzymes slightly differ in physicochemical characteristics and specificity of action, but their properties are generally quite similar.

Bromelain is the common name for enzymes found in various plants of the *Bromeliaceae* family. It is a mixture of eight high-molecular-weight glycoproteins — cysteine proteases. Bromelain from pineapple stems is the most studied, and some amounts of these enzymes are present in leaves and fruits (both green and ripe). The enzymes **ananain** and **comosain** are also found in pineapple.

In modern enzymatic peel formulations, **ficin** (obtained from the milky sap of the fig tree *Ficuscarica*), **actinidain** (from kiwi), **aleurain** (from barley), as well as proteases from mango, pumpkin, yam, and other plants are used.

In papaya, pineapple, and some other plants, in addition to proteases, other enzymes are present — amylases (amylolytic enzymes that hydrolyze α-(1,4)-glycoside bond in amylose, amylopectin, glycogen, and other maltooligosaccharides), lysozyme (a hydrolase that breaks down bacterial walls), and lipases (involved in the breakdown of fats, which are esters of glycerol and higher fatty acids). Plant lipases are mainly found in seeds, fruits, tubers, rhizomes of cereals, crucifers, and legumes. Lipases have been found in papaya and pineapple. When skin peels based on the so-called plant "pulp" are applied to the skin, the lipase contained in it works synergistically with proteases, destroying intercellular lipids of the *stratum corneum* and allowing proteases to penetrate deeper into the *stratum corneum*. Lysozyme, at the same time, provides antibacterial skin protection.

Nowadays, **enzymes of microbial origin** are typically included in skincare products. Microbial proteases belong to the class of **serine proteases**. Their active center contains the amino acid serine.

It should be noted that the activity and diversity of bacterial proteases are much higher than that of plant proteases. This is because proteases are the main survival tool for microbes, a means of invasion into the host tissues, and spreading throughout the body. In addition, there are as many hosts as there are specific conditions to which they need to adapt. Therefore, one such enzyme, **subtilisin (subtilopeptidase)**, a metabolic product of *Bacillus subtilis*, acts less specifically than papain, breaking down more diverse proteins, and is consequently more effective at removing protein contaminants. The U.S. Food and Drug Administration (FDA) has declared isolated and purified subtilisin safe for use in food, detergents, and cosmetic products.

Different strains of *Bacillus subtilis* and some other microorganisms are used to produce subtilisin, and the technology of isolation, purification, and stabilization of the enzyme also varies from manufacturer to manufacturer. Therefore, the resulting enzyme products are not identical in properties. Each manufacturer gives its product a unique brand name to distinguish it from its counterparts. It is not yet a ready-to-use product but rather a single component incorporated into a cosmetic product.

For example, an enzyme product called **travase** (Travase®) is included in topical medicinal products for clearing of wound scabs — such preparations are used in anti-burn therapy.

Keratoline (Keratoline®) is another subtilisin-based product adapted for use in skincare products. It has subtilisin dissolved in a liquid aqueous gel with a small amount of glycerin and propylene glycol to stabilize the enzyme and facilitate its introduction into the complex composition.

Proteases of animal origin can be found in cosmetic peels: aspartate proteases — **pepsin** and serine proteases — **trypsin**, **chymotrypsin**, and **pancreatin**. However, the general trend away from using ingredients of animal origin in favor of biotechnological and plant-based components, and the lower stability of animal proteases, have led to their gradual removal from cosmetic formulations.

As for the well-known collagenase, it is successfully used in medicine for debridement — removal of tissue decay products from wounds. Treating wounds with proteolytic enzymes accelerates healing, preventing infection and the formation of rough scars. It is noteworthy that, for wounds, the drug is applied to the skin deprived of its barrier, which means that the penetration through the *stratum corneum* is not an issue. We do not know of any approved peeling/exfoliation product that contains this enzyme.

There are also **modified natural peptidases**. Modified enzymes are more stable than natural ones. For example, cross-linked papain (cross-papain) was developed by specialists at BASF. The individual molecules of the enzyme are cross-linked with a heat-stable crosslinking agent so that their active centers remain available for reaction with the substrate. Such an aggregate of several enzyme units is attached to a polymer substrate. The result is a complex with high enzymatic activity immersed in sodium alginate gel for additional stabilization.

Cross-papain withstands high temperatures, and its individual enzyme units become resistant even to surfactants, which makes it possible to include cross-papain in emulsions. This is a great advantage because naturally unmodified proteases can only be incorporated into aqueous solutions or gels that do not contain emulsifiers.

Making a valid formulation containing enzymes is not easy. One problem is that proteolytic enzymes are protein compounds, and in an aqueous solution, they can serve as a substrate for each other (i.e., one enzyme molecule can cleave another enzyme molecule). Therefore, as a rule, the proteolytic activity of the enzyme components decreases markedly or even disappears completely in the process of making a cosmetic product. This problem can be solved by chemically modifying the enzymes, e.g., by "attaching" propylene glycol or dextran to their protein chain. The modified enzyme retains its activity in an aqueous solution for a long time. Another way to preserve the enzyme activity is using two-component preparations consisting of dry lyophilized enzyme powder and an activating solution. Since the enzyme is dissolved directly on the skin, its activity is preserved.

Another problem is the risk of skin damage from prolonged contact with proteolytic (protein-dissolving) enzymes. Therefore, these enzymes are usually added only to preparations that need to be washed off the skin.

Indications for enzymatic peeling are:
- Scaling
- Acne (non-inflammatory) and post-acne
- Seborrheic dermatitis
- Pigmentation disorders

Contraindications:
- Contact dermatitis
- Photodermatoses
- Individual intolerance to the components of the peel formulation
- Acne or chronic dermatoses in the acute stage

The exposure time does not exceed 30 minutes, after which the preparation is thoroughly washed off with plenty of warm water or removed with wet wipes. The enzymatic peeling can be performed 1–2 times every 7–14 days.

Among the **possible complications** are rarely observed allergic dermatitis, acne exacerbation, and seborrheic dermatitis. People with a history of allergy (including latex allergy) must be treated with caution before prescribing the enzymatic peel. It is necessary to test the preparation by putting a small amount on the skin at the bend of the elbow.

An enzymatic peeling would be more accurately called an enzymatic exfoliation because, in fact, it removes only the very top corneocytes

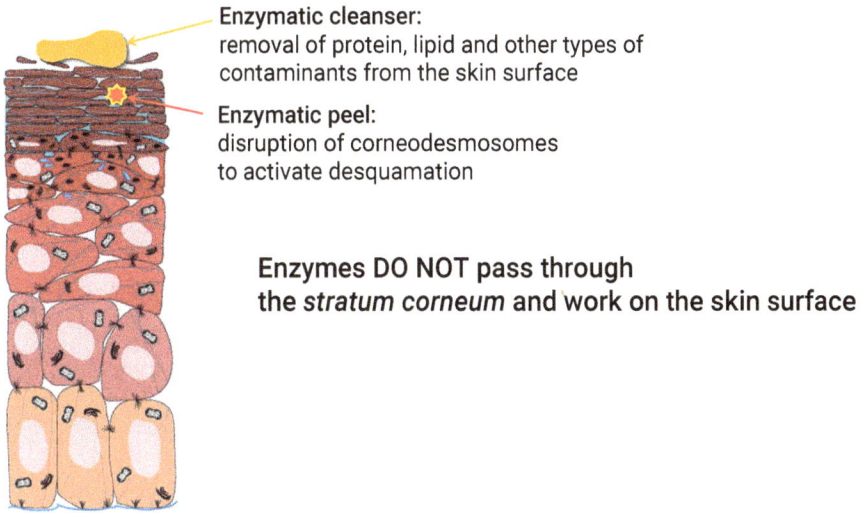

Enzymatic cleanser:
removal of protein, lipid and other types of contaminants from the skin surface

Enzymatic peel:
disruption of corneodesmosomes to activate desquamation

Enzymes DO NOT pass through the *stratum corneum* and work on the skin surface

Figure II-2-4. Targets for enzymatic peels and cleansers

and protein impurities from the skin surface (**Fig. II-2-4**). Although enzymatic peeling is also used as an independent procedure, its use in the preparatory stage is the most logical because it does not have such a strong exfoliating effect as other peeling agents. However, it successfully solves the problem of smoothing the *stratum corneum*, increasing its permeability, and softening the heads of comedones. That is why we consider it here and not in the section on treatments with intensive influence, although, we repeat, in some skincare procedures, enzymatic preparations are used as the main means of intensive influence.

Enzymatic peels have also proven their worth in in-home care. Studies have shown that regular use of preparations with proteolytic enzymes for 8–12 weeks leads to a significant improvement in skin structure, comparable to the effects of a single peel with high AHA concentration.

2.5.3. Physical treatment

Although we review the cosmetic products used to care for healthy skin in this book, it is important to say a few words about the physical methods available to most professionals and used for exfoliation in many skincare programs.

Desincrustation

Desincrustation (synonym: electro peeling) is a physical method based on electroplating with an alkaline solution designed to cleanse the facial skin. Aggregates of sebum, makeup, and dust are not water-soluble, so it is difficult to remove them from the surface of the skin and hair follicles. Disinfection is accomplished through a chemical reaction called "saponification," in which fatty acids from sebum secretions react with alkalis, resulting in soaps that are easily washed away and removed from the skin surface.

Desincrustation is thus used to treat oily skin with excess sebum secretion (forehead, nose, chin) to soften sebaceous plugs (saponification of comedones). In addition, exposure to electric current promotes the removal of sebaceous gland secretions from the pores, increases vascular permeability, and causes hydration of the cells.

Ultrasonic peeling

One way to break the bonds between the corneocytes and accelerate exfoliation is to use intense ultrasound waves to cavitate the contact medium applied to the skin. This, in turn, leads to the destruction of corneodesmosomes, which accelerates desquamation. Ultrasound also affects the dermis, especially its dense fibrous structures, "loosening" and accelerating their renewal. The lifting effect observed after the ultrasound procedure is thought to be primarily due to increased *stratum corneum* hydration, probably due to the depolymerization of hyaluronic and chondroitin acids.

The indications for ultrasonic peeling are moderate age-related keratosis and superficial wrinkles in cheeks, eye corners, and chin. In case of hyperkeratosis, seborrhea, or inflammatory processes, ultrasonic peeling is not recommended.

It is important to note that ultrasonic peeling is very gentle and is much gentler than microdermabrasion. It "works" by peeling the uppermost layers of the skin. The procedure frequency depends on the skin's age and condition. It is enough for young patients with non-problem skin to do an ultrasonic peel once a month as a preventive monoprocedure. In the case of propensity toward comedone formation ultrasonic peeling can be combined with a superficial chemical peeling in a special course (once every one or two weeks, a course of

4–6–8 treatments). Such a course is designed for the initial stage of seborrhea/acne formation or as a maintenance therapy when there is no need to mechanically clean the skin. For "old" comedones, ultrasound peeling can help loosen and soften them to facilitate manual removal later, but it cannot remove them and heal the skin. So, when a patient has already formed acne, it is too late to cleanse, and treatment should be initiated immediately.

Often the accumulation of corneocytes makes the skin look gray and dull. An ultrasonic peeling is effective in superficial exfoliation, as the skin becomes pinkish and looks fresh and rested after the procedure. If the skin has aesthetic defects like spots, comedones, or inflammatory elements that cannot be eliminated quickly, more "serious" exposure methods are necessary.

In the older age group, ultrasonic peeling is usually used when the patient does not want to perform chemical peeling or mesotherapy/biorevitalization and prefers a delicate treatment. In such cases, ultrasonic peeling is recommended as a variant of light cleansing and micro-massage. Massage results in a slight pink blush due to the vasodilatation in the treated area. Certain limitations arise in this regard. Namely, if the patient has couperosis, it is better not to apply ultrasound to the affected skin, as it can cause the blood vessels to dilate, aggravating the couperosis.

The combination of superficial chemical exfoliation and ultrasound peeling is ideal for clients who do not want their skin to peel, as most dead cells are removed during the procedure. Combining these methods, as opposed to traditionally using them separately, can improve the skin appearance much faster, reducing the course to six treatments at two-week intervals. However, one should not expect significant smoothing of skin microrelief in case of post-acne scars or significant lightening of pigmentation, as this requires more aggressive and deep action, and the ultrasonic peeling effect is limited to the *stratum corneum*.

2.6. Moisturizing as the final stage of skin preparation for an intensive treatment

An important task in preparation of the skin for the subsequent intensive intervention is a temporary increase of permeability of its barrier structures. After the removal of external "barriers" (impurities, corneocyte masses), which are obstacles on the path to the *stratum corneum*, we can proceed to weaken the "fortress wall" — the lipid barrier that cements the corneocytes and does not let almost anything through the *stratum corneum*.

We have repeatedly stated that **one of the most effective ways to weaken the barrier is hyperhydration**. Increasing the water content of the *stratum corneum* above the normal level causes disorganization of the intercellular lipid layers, and the lipid barrier becomes more permeable.

After cleansing and exfoliation, the *stratum corneum* is **supersaturated** with water-based preparations — most often, toners are used for this purpose, so this step is called toning in many professional procedures. Various solutions and serums can also be used.

Initially, toners were used to rinse away residual alkaline cleansers from the skin and "extinguish" them by restoring the skin's surface pH to a more acidic range. Nowadays, however, there is no need for this since most modern cleansers are weakly acidic; still, it is important to rinse surfactants well.

Various biologically active compounds can be added to tonics. For example, glycerin, hyaluronic acid, butylene glycol, and various oils and silicones are added in order to further increase their moisturizing potential. Fruit acids are also included (see above) — such products are often referred to as "light peels" or "exfoliating lotions," although using them in the procedure does not lead to exfoliation as such but moisturizes the skin well.

Preparations may contain anti-inflammatory and soothing components (most often of plant origin — extracts of green tea, chamomile, and grape seed) and cooling substances (menthol).

Serums typically have increased concentrations of polymers (hyaluronic acid, polyethylene glycols) and glycerol as structure-forming agents. The solutions do not contain any gel-forming agents, but they include water-soluble humectants — amino acids, urea, lactic acid, sodium pyroglutamate, and mineral salts.

2.7. Seasonal skin cleansing

The choice of cleansing methods and specific preparations is guided not only by the skin's condition but also by the climatic conditions. Studies show that people who live permanently in dry and hot climates tend to have a more developed epidermal barrier than those who live in humid areas. This distinction has emerged because in a dry environment, the skin synthesizes epidermal lipids more actively and renews its barrier structures faster than when it is in a humid environment. Consequently, skin preparation in dry regions should involve softening and thinning the *stratum corneum*. In the absence of contraindications, the preparation choice for the professional procedure is a scrub. In wet weather, preference should be given to milder enzymatic preparations.

In summer, the skin usually produces more sebum and sweat, so it needs to be cleaned more thoroughly. In winter, the synthesis of ceramides and other epidermal barrier lipids in the skin decreases, which promotes skin dryness and weakens the epidermal barrier. Meanwhile, people with sensitive skin usually report increased sensitivity in the summertime. If you have sensitive skin, use only mild cleansers and not scrubs.

Cleansing the skin and smoothing the *stratum corneum* is the first step in preparing the skin for cosmetic treatments. However, cleansing usually destroys the skin's acid mantle and weakens the epidermal barrier, which can provoke irritation during the subsequent intensive care phase. Ideally, skin preparations should dissolve and remove sebum, makeup, and sweat, exfoliate and remove the top layers of the *stratum corneum* to smooth it out, intensely moisturize the skin to increase permeability, and, if necessary, soothe the skin before aggressive cosmetic procedures are performed.

Part III

Special skincare products and treatments

After the *stratum corneum* has been cleaned and its permeability temporarily increased, intensive treatment to solve specific problems begins.

In fact, for the skin, an aesthetic defect like pigmented spot, wrinkle, or even scar is not a problem because it does not prevent the skin from performing its functions. Therefore, the skin simply does not notice such issues and does nothing to get rid of them. To get the skin out of the equilibrium, you need a jolt that forces it to change. In structural renewal, the aesthetic defect can shrink or even disappear entirely and be replaced by normal tissue.

Regardless of the problem to be solved, all modern skincare means of intensive influence are divided into two groups:

- Negative stimulation methods
- Positive stimulation methods

The principle of **negative stimulation** is used by methods that trigger the renewal processes by destroying specific skin structures or suppressing certain processes. If we talk specifically about cosmetic products, this group includes preparations for chemical peels based on keratolytics, proteolytic enzymes, and hydroxy acids, destroying the barrier structures of the skin and thus giving a signal for the cellular renewal of the epidermis. This group also includes depigmenting agents that inhibit the process of melanogenesis by suppressing its individual stages. Negative stimulation is a necessary step in the treatment of unaesthetic-looking formations on the skin such as scars, pigment spots, keratosis plaques, papillomas, and warts.

Positive stimulation activates specific processes in the skin without destroying or suppressing them. Retinoids, synthetic peptides–biomimetics, and some components of plant extracts carry out positive stimulation. It is used to restore disturbed equilibrium (homeostasis), prevention of potential issues, and skin improvement.

Methods of positive and negative stimulation are often combined within a course, as, for example, in the elimination of post-acne scars, when it is necessary to destroy defective structures as well as stimulate the formation of healthy tissue.

In this part, we look at the cosmetic products used for the active treatment of specific skin problems.

Chapter 1
Chemical peels

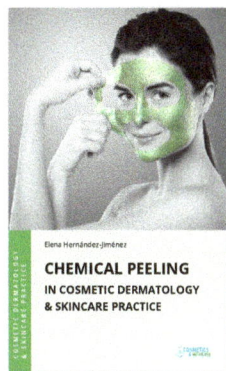

Chemical peeling as an active topical treatment is explained in detail in the *Chemical Peeling in Cosmetic Dermatology & Skincare Practice* book. In this book, we discuss the main points to consider when working with this method.

1.1. Indications and contraindications

Currently, chemical peels are used to solve aesthetic problems of **epidermal origin**, i.e., those that emerged due to changes in the epidermis. Epidermal problems can be divided into two main groups.

1. **Textural changes** associated with impaired keratinization: surface wrinkles, roughness, roughness
2. **Color changes** associated with impaired pigment formation and lipofuscin accumulation in cells: dyschromia (hypo- or hyperpigmentation, dullness, tint — yellowish, reddish, grayish)

In the pathogenesis and clinical picture of many skin conditions or even pathologies, several epidermal problems are often present simultaneously (**Fig. III-1-1**), which is the indication for using chemical peels.

For example, in the case of **post-acne**, pigmentation disorders and altered topography are observed. Keratosis, uneven tone, and superficial wrinkles are the **skin-aging** signs. Pigmentation disorders and coarsening are characteristic of the skin **photodamage**. Pathologies such as actinic keratosis, age-related lentigo, and *pseudofolliculitis barbae* have disorders of keratinization and hyperkeratosis in their pathogenesis. **Table III-1-1** shows the general indications for the chemical peel procedure.

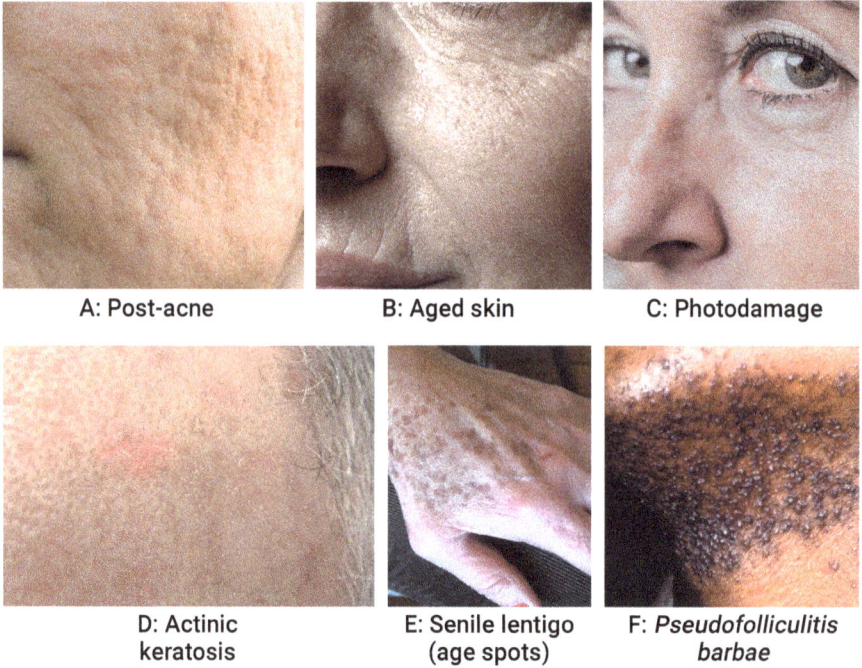

A: Post-acne B: Aged skin C: Photodamage

D: Actinic keratosis E: Senile lentigo (age spots) F: *Pseudofolliculitis barbae*

Figure III-1-1. General indications for chemical peeling (Images by Freepik [A–C] and Wikipedia [D–F])

Table III-1-1. Main indications for chemical peeling in different life stages

UP TO 25 YEARS	25–30 YEARS	30 YEARS AND OLDER
• Acne (non-inflammatory) • Sebum excess and enlarged pores (oily skin) • Skin with consequences of previous acne (scarring, pigment spots) • Uneven pigmentation	• Elimination of the consequences of previously suffered acne (post-acne) • Prevention of skin aging • Actinic dermatitis • Hyperpigmentation	• Prevention and treatment of aesthetic defects (wrinkles, folds, withering skin) • Hyperpigmentation of various etiologies • Keratosis • Prevention and treatment of papillomavirus infection • Preparation for dermabrasion and plastic surgery

Today, chemical peeling is successfully included in a comprehensive framework of cosmetic treatments and is combined with injection and physical methods that ensure the impact on deep structures, achieving excellent results with minimal risk.

Skin inflammation (even the lightest!) is an absolute contraindication for chemical peeling. It can be caused by various factors (disease, infection, trauma), but if it is present, chemical peeling should not be performed in the inflamed area.

Peeling is contraindicated in cases of **skin hypersensitivity**, as well as **individual intolerance** to the substances contained in the preparation.

In addition, each type of peeling has its own list of contraindications. We discuss this list in the chapter on the specific peeling.

1.2. Biological basis

1.2.1. Peeling is based on the skin's capacity for self-renewal

Normally, the division rate of basal keratinocytes is equal to the rate of desquamation of corneocytes. A complete replacement of keratinocytes in the epidermis takes 28 days on average (**physiological regeneration**). However, in damaged skin, the number of cell mitoses in the basal layer increases, the newly formed keratinocytes start moving up and sideways faster, and their maturation processes are also accelerated because the skin has to close the "gap in the barrier" as soon as possible (**physiological repair**).

Epidermal regeneration and repair have much in common. They are realized due to the genetic program determining changes (differentiation) of a keratinocyte's life path, which begins in the basal layer and ends in the *stratum corneum*.

Any effect on the skin that aims at structural reorganization must rely on the skin's capacity for self-renewal.

The deeper the lesion, the greater the load on the skin's repair systems and the greater the chance that something in the repair process can go wrong. Although a more aggressive peeling may seem able to achieve more significant skin regeneration, before choosing it, you should assess the risks and try to match the depth of damage to the repairing capabilities of the skin. For example, the older a person is, the poorer their repair systems are, so we should be more cautious about procedures that damage the skin. The same applies to people suffering from a somatic disease or in an unstable psychoemotional state — their resistance to aggressive external factors is reduced, and recovery resources are depleted.

1.2.2. Epidermis, the main target for chemical peels

The first question the skincare practitioner must answer before starting the chemical peeling is: what exactly and how much should be destroyed?

The main impact of chemical peeling is on the epidermis, which is understandable because it is where the peel is applied. Above all, the chemical substances react with the epidermal structures. The echoes of these reactions reach the dermal layer, which, in turn, reacts to them (or does not react). Still, these are only echoes of the processes unfolding in the epidermis because the main targets for chemical peeling agents are located directly in it.

Peels' active components penetrate to different depths and interact with the skin structures differently. All peeling agents used today, except retinol, "work" through damage — directly destroying their target or disrupting its functioning. For these substances, the following statement is true: the deeper the targets are, the more serious the trauma caused to the skin during the procedure.

The following **factors determine the degree of skin damage** during chemical peeling:
- Chemical nature of the peeling agent
- Concentration of the peeling agent
- pH value of the applied preparation (for acid peels)

- Carrier, i.e., those substances that are contained in the peel preparation and that affect the rate of penetration of the peeling agent through the *stratum corneum*
- Exposure time
- Initial condition of the skin on which the peeling preparation is applied

According to the **depth**:

1. **Exfoliation** (the most superficial peeling) — accelerating the exfoliation of the most superficial corneocytes, which are ready to leave the skin, but still remain on its surface, for example, because of the mixture of sebum, dust, and cosmetics sticking them together (often exfoliation is performed in the first — preparatory — stage of cosmetic treatment).
2. **Superficial peeling** — action at the level of the *stratum corneum* (disintegration of corneodesmosomes, changes in the activity of enzymes involved in the formation of the lipid barrier, and proteolytic destruction of corneodesmosomes).
3. **Medium-depth peeling** — damaging effect up to the level of the granular layer of the epidermis.
4. **Medium-depth/deep peeling** — damaging effect up to the basal layer of the epidermis.
5. **Deep peeling** is a skin injury resulting in the removal of the epidermis, part of the growth zone, and the top layers of the dermis that protrude into the epidermis.

The safest action is within the *stratum corneum* — dull corneocytes and the dirt adhering to them are scrubbed off, the skin surface is smoothed, and the underlying living cells of the epidermis are unaffected. Often such polishing is enough to noticeably refresh the skin and give it a healthy and beautiful shine. If the action is at the level of the *stratum corneum* (exfoliation and superficial peeling) and/or proceeds without damaging living cells (retinol peeling), it is a cosmetic procedure that is one of the stages of skincare routine and/or serves to prepare the skin for a further stronger peeling and can be performed both in the salon and at home.

If the chemical peeling damages living cells, such a procedure is classified as medical and must be performed in a medical facility.

Pain, swelling, long recovery time, unwanted reactions in the form of pigmentation disorders, and unpredictability, in general, are the characteristics of the deep peel procedure, which is inevitably accompanied by severe damage to the epidermal barrier. Fortunately, today we have an excellent alternative for working with deep skin structures in injectable and physical methods that minimize or do not traumatize at all.

1.2.3. Peeling "outside-in" and peeling "inside-out": what's the difference?

Some time after the peeling procedure, the skin begins to peel. The nature of peeling (e.g., the onset and duration of the active peeling phase, the scales size and shape, the peeling intensity) depends on:

- Degree of skin damage
- Chemical nature of the peeling agent
- Initial condition of the skin
- General state of client's health

We have already mentioned that skin exfoliation occurs because of the continuous natural change of the epidermis cellular composition, but if the skin is healthy, we do not notice the exfoliation.

Visible scaling is a universal skin response to damage. Damaged skin tries to get rid of destroyed elements as soon as possible — it sheds them off, making room for new, functionally active ones. It is through damage that peeling agents such as phenol, trichloroacetic acid (TCA), salicylic acids, and proteolytic enzymes act. **Peels performed through destabilizing effects on the *stratum corneum* are called "outside-in" peels.**

However, skin desquamation can be caused not only by damaging its barrier structures. Recall that the rate of division of basal keratinocytes is normally related to the corneocyte exfoliation rate. If the rate of division is increased by stimulating mitosis, the newly formed cells start to move to the surface faster, as if displacing the overlying cell layers; eventually, there is a mass reset of corneocytes on top, which is visible to the naked eye. This is how retinol, which is also used as a peeling agent, works. **Retinol triggers desquamation by stimulat-**

OUTSIDE-IN	INSIDE-OUT

Exfoliation through destraction or inhibition			Exfoliation through stimulation
Proteins' denaturation	Corneodesmosomes' hydrolysis	Changes in the activity of the *stratum corneum'* enzymes	Activation of basal keratinocyte proliferation and migration

- Phenol
- TCA
- Resorcinol
- Salicylic acid
- LHA

- Proteolytic enzymes

- AHAs
- PHAs

- Retinol
- Retinyl esters

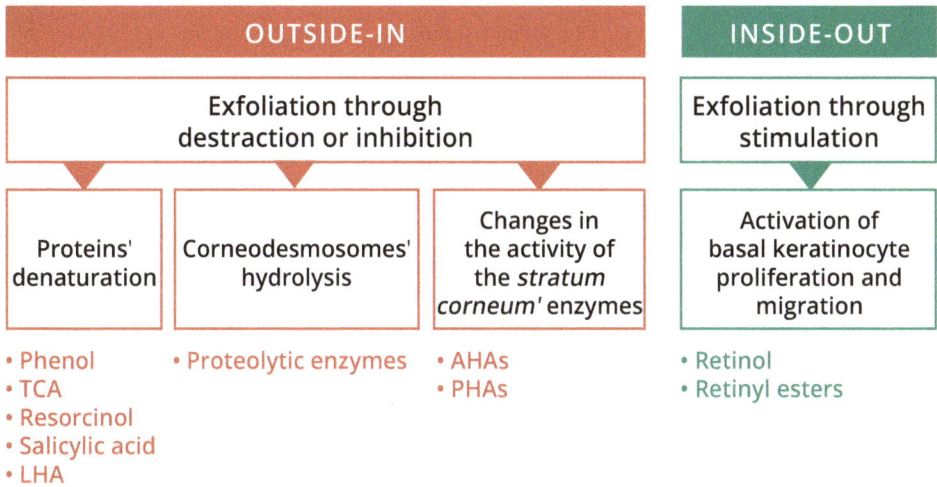

Figure III-1-2. Chemical peeling "outside-in" and "inside-out": the principle of action and peeling agents

ing the division of basal keratinocytes. And because the *stratum corneum* itself does not react in any way to retinol, retinol peels are called "inside-out" peels.

According to this principle, all currently known peeling agents are divided into two groups: **destroyers** and **stimulators** (**Fig. III-1-2**).

Peeling agents differ in their chemical nature and mechanisms of action. There are four main types of chemical peel formulations:

1. Keratolytic peels
2. Acid peels
3. Enzymatic peels
4. Retinol peels

Although they are all peels, peeling agents are not interchangeable. Each type of chemical peel is unique in what it does best or only does. Let's take a closer look at the main features of each type of peel.

1.3. Keratolytic peels

Keratolytic peels were the first to appear on the market. Phenol, TCA, salicylic acid, and resorcinol have been used to remove scars and age spots since the 1880s. The term "keratolytic" was coined to describe these compounds, which means "dissolver of corneocytes" (from the Greek κέρατο — horn). This name was given because, when keratolytic substances came into contact with the skin, a whitish plaque appeared on the surface, which was then easily washed off. Most of the plaque is made up of modified corneocytes filled with keratin. But keratin is not the only target for keratolytics, so in addition to exfoliating, they have other effects.

1.3.1. Mechanism of action

Keratolytics react chemically with proteins and **break the disulfide bonds** formed between the sulfur atoms of the amino acid cysteine. With the help of disulfide bonds, the protein (or protein complex if it has several chains) maintains the necessary configuration in space — such a protein is called **native**, and only in this form it is capable of performing the functions assigned to it, whether structural, enzymatic, or otherwise. As a result of breaking the stabilizing bonds, the protein unfolds and turns into an amino acid chain — a denatured protein that is no longer active (**Fig. III–1-3**).

Keratolytics interact with all proteins having disulfide bonds, i.e., their action is not selective and is not limited to keratin. In addition to keratin, other proteins in the *stratum corneum* and epidermis will also be denatured when encountering a keratolytic, affecting the clinical result.

NATIVE PROTEIN   DENATURED PROTEIN

S–S-bonds

*Unfolding
protein chain*

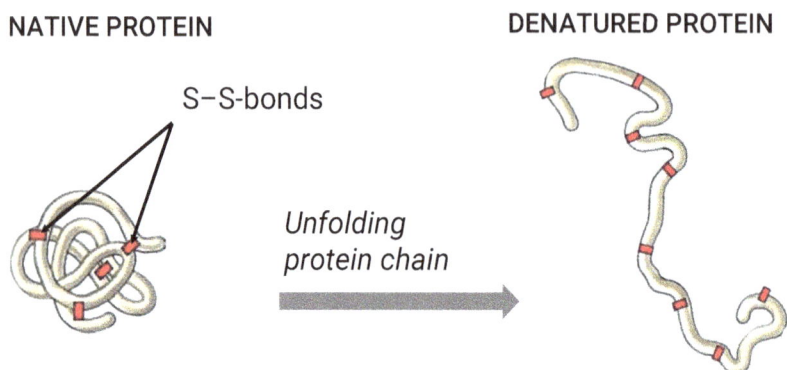

Figure III-1-3. Mechanism of keratolytic action: breaking of stabilizing disulfide bonds (–S–S–) in a protein molecule or a protein complex

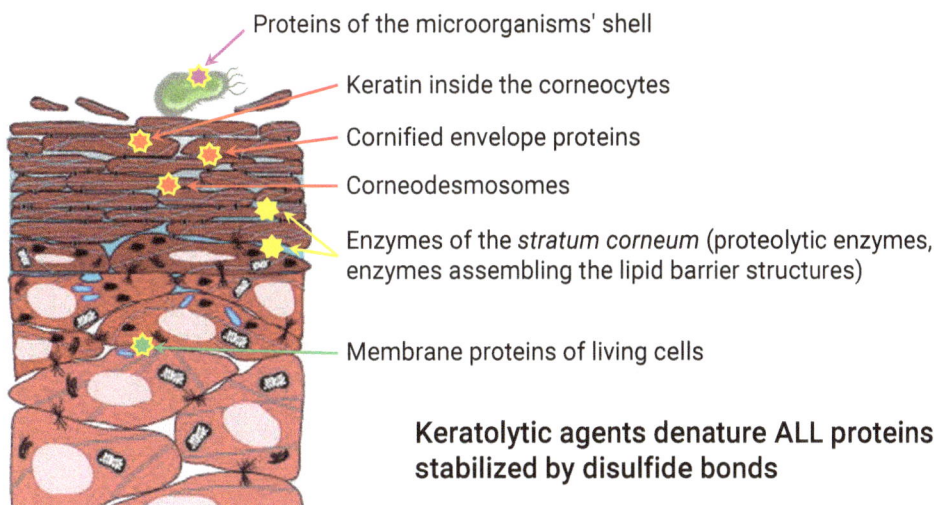

Proteins of the microorganisms' shell

Keratin inside the corneocytes

Cornified envelope proteins

Corneodesmosomes

Enzymes of the *stratum corneum* (proteolytic enzymes, enzymes assembling the lipid barrier structures)

Membrane proteins of living cells

Keratolytic agents denature ALL proteins stabilized by disulfide bonds

Figure III-1-4. Targets for keratolytic agents

In the *stratum corneum*, the keratolytic targets are (**Fig. III-1-4**):

- Corneocyte-associated proteins — **keratin** (inside) and **cornified envelope proteins**
- **Corneodesmosomes** — protein bridges that bind corneocytes together and maintain the integrity of the *stratum corneum*
- *Stratum corneum*'s **enzymes** — proteolytic enzymes (they cut the corneodesmosomes and are responsible for desquamation) and enzymes responsible for the assembly of the lipid barrier located between the corneocytes

What happens if the substance passes through the *stratum corneum* and ends up in the territory of living cells? The keratolytic reacts chemically with the proteins, damaging their structure. A person feels **pain** when a keratolytic enters the epidermis because these substances denaturate membrane proteins of the skin receptors. But in this book, we will not address phenol and TCA — these substances can cause significant trauma and their use is currently banned (although TCA is still used in various formulations, despite restrictions). Briefly, the keratolytics that are approved for use are salicylic acid, liposalicylic acid, and resorcinol.

1.3.2. Keratolytic substances

Salicylic acid and liposalicylic acid

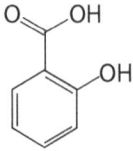

Salicylic acid (2-hydroxybenzoic acid; $C_6H_4(OH)COOH$) is a colorless crystalline substance, well soluble in ethanol, diethyl ether, and other polar organic solvents, but is poorly soluble in water (1.8 g/l at 20°C).

Salicylic acid was first isolated from the bark of willow (*Salix L.*), where its name comes from, and it has also been found in other plants, such as birch bark and gaultheria leaves.

Salicylic acid is a phenol to which a carboxy group was added. The result is a molecule with a hydroxy and a carboxy group. It is by this formal attribute that salicylic acid is classified as a hydroxy acid. However, chemically, this is incorrect because, in the salicylic acid molecule, both functional groups (carboxylic and hydroxyl) are attached directly to the benzene ring, not to the hydrocarbon chain. This confuses skincare practitioners and customers, who put salicylic acid on par with glycolic, lactic, tartaric, and other AHAs. The chemical properties of salicylic acid have nothing in common with water-soluble AHAs, and it is not even correct to classify it as β-hydroxy acid.

In contact with the skin, salicylic acid quickly reacts with the proteins of the *stratum corneum*, primary with the corneodesmosomes and proteins of the cornified envelopes. It destroys them and provokes **rapid desquamation** of corneocytes. During the procedure, we see a white plaque (frost) and coarse scaling. The skin becomes loose, and its permeability increases.

The **antiseptic effect** also appears immediately after applying the substance to the skin and is explained by the fact that salicylic acid denatures the proteins of the shells of all microorganisms in the treatment area.

But **delayed desquamation** is not always present (**Fig. III-1-5**). It is associated with damage to the *stratum corneum*'s enzymes responsible for its formation and renewal. If the enzymes are disrupted, the structures that are currently in the depth of the *stratum corneum* are not correct — the skin tends to "drop" them as soon as possible.

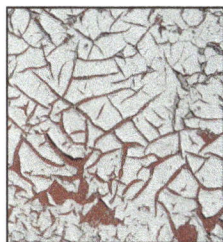

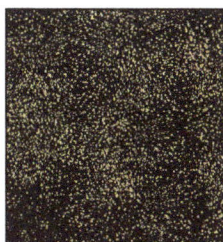

	Frost Large flakes Permeability increase
	Fine flakes (possible)
	Antiseptic
	Reduction of skin oiliness

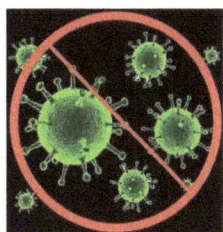

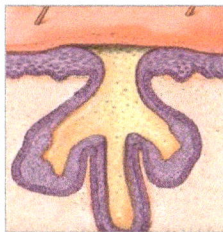

Figure III-1-5. Clinical effects of salicylic peeling

Fine flaking a few days after salicylic peeling is just a sign of such enzyme failure. However, this is not always the case and is usually related to the exposure time — the longer it is, the more likely it is that the salicylic acid will disrupt the enzymes.

All these are nonspecific effects, typical of keratolytics in general. Apart from these, salicylic acid has a very important **specific effect**: being small and fat-soluble, it penetrates sebaceous glands filled with sebum quite easily, reaches sebocytes, and suppresses sebum production. Moreover, it triggers the death of sebocytes through apoptosis, reducing the number of secretory cells in the sebaceous glands, which reduces the amount of sebum produced. Recent studies have shed light on another known observation — it relates to the anti-inflammatory effect of salicylic drugs. It turned out that among the cytokines that sebocytes release, pro-inflammatory mediators trigger and maintain inflammation, and salicylic acid suppresses their production.

Salicylic acid is often included in skincare products for oily skin. Due to its keratolytic action, it opens comedones, improving the sebum evacuation from the sebaceous gland ducts. The average concentration of salicylic acid is as follows:

- in skincare products: 0.5–1% (in some cases up to 2%)
- in masks: 2–5%
- in peel products: 15–30%

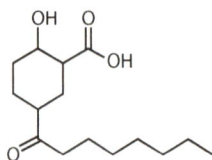

Liposalicylic acid (LHA) is 2-hydroxy-5-octanoylbenzoic acid (C8-β-lipohydroxy acid), a salicylic acid molecule to which a fatty acid is attached. It is well soluble in fats while being insoluble in water.

A lipid derivative of salicylic acid, **lipohydroxy acid (LHA)**, is known on the cosmetic market. The LHA molecule is larger and has a higher affinity to lipids, so it accumulates in the lipid layer of the *stratum corneum* and loosens it.

Studies have shown that salicylic acid and LHA destroy corneodesmosomes differently. Salicylic acid is active throughout the entire thickness of the *stratum corneum*, while LHA acts on the corneocytes located at a depth of the 3rd–4th layers. It is at this depth that the desquamation process begins. Unlike salicylic acid, which acts on any corneodesmosomes, LHA selectively affects only those that have already begun to undergo the process of enzymatic destruction. Finally, the very nature of the destruction of corneodesmosomes in LHA differs from that of salicylic acid: in the case of LHA, the protein bridges are more severely destroyed.

Additionally, LHA exhibits antimicrobial, fungicidal, anti-inflammatory, and comedolytic properties, making this substance an effective component for light peels, skincare products for oily skin, acne and post-acne treatments, and restoration of photodamaged skin. The concentration of LHA in in-home peel products is 5–10%. The valid patent for this substance belongs to L'Oréal, so now it is found only in the products of this company's brands.

Salicylic acid and LHA combine well with other peeling agents, acting synergistically with them. By gently exfoliating the *stratum corneum*, they indirectly stimulate the division of basal keratinocytes. They are characterized by a high level of safety and are well tolerated, even by sensitive skin. As a rule, the effects of salicylic acid and LHA are cumulative and require several treatments with products containing these compounds.

Salicylic peeling should be used to treat signs of chrono- and photoaging if the skin is not deficient in sebum. Preparations with salicylic acid (whether for care or for peeling) are contraindicated for low-sebum skin. Accordingly, to treat epidermal age-related changes in dry, low-sebum skin, one should choose enzymatic or acidic peel.

The anti-inflammatory effects of salicylic acid, supported by antiseptic, comedolytic, and anti-keratosis effects, allow us to specifically recommend salicylic peeling for seborrhea and skin pathologies associated with increased sebum production (acne, seborrheic dermatitis, seborrheic keratosis), as well as for psoriasis.

Indications for salicylic peeling:
- Epidermal age-related changes
- Photoaging
- Oily skin
- Acne (non-inflammatory)
- Post-acne
- Seborrheic dermatitis
- Psoriasis (psoriatic lesions)
- Seborrheic keratosis (seborrheic keratoma, blue warts)

Contraindications:
- Decreased sebaceous gland activity (low-sebum skin)
- Atopic dermatitis
- Herpes in the active phase or with a recent exacerbation
- Hypersensitivity to salicylic acid
- Allergies to aspirin and salicylates
- Sunburns in the intended treatment area
- Pregnancy, lactation
- A laser or IPL treatment within the last two weeks

Salicylic peeling is a superficial treatment that patients with any skin phototype tolerate well. A course usually includes 5–10 sessions at 7–14-day intervals. A skincare practitioner with a paramedical background can perform salicylic peeling. Cosmetic products with salicylic acid can be used 1–2 times a day.

Resorcinol and Jessner peel

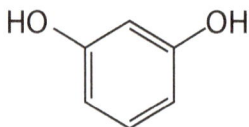

Resorcinol (resorcinol, 1,3-dihydroxybenzene, meta-dihydroxybenzene, $C_6H_4(OH)_2$) has the physical appearance of colorless crystals with a peculiar odor. The structure is like hydroquinone, differing only by the position of hydroxyl groups.

Resorcinol is also a derivative of phenol, which is much less common than salicylic acid because of its higher irritant potential.

In dermatology, resorcinol became known thanks to the American physician Max Jessner, who included it along with salicylic acid in a remedy to remove hyperkeratotic epidermal lesions. This remedy is now known as a **Jessner peel**. It is used not only for localized cauterization but also to even out wrinkles and overall skin tone to rejuvenate or treat post-acne scars. The classic peel contains the following ingredients: salicylic acid — 14%, resorcinol — 14%, lactic acid —14%, and 95% ethanol solution — up to 100 ml.

Ethanol is alcohol, a universal organic solvent that dissolves water and fat equally well. Ethanol quickly dissolves the hydrolipidic mantle and penetrates the *stratum corneum*'s intercellular spaces, disrupting the lipid barrier. This means that salicylic acid and resorcinol can more easily pass through the *stratum corneum* and get near the living cells of the epidermis faster.

Lactic acid is designed to soften the effect of the two keratolytic agents and the organic solvent on the skin. But the formula composition is still quite aggressive. If applied in several layers and the exposure time is relatively long, damage at the level of the living layers of the epidermis occurs.

The Jessner peeling, as well as the salicylic peeling, should not be performed on low-sebum skin. The list of **contraindications for Jessner peels** is broader than for salicylic peels and includes the following conditions or diseases (Grimes P. E., 2006):
- Low-sebum skin (e.g., age-related, atopic)
- Purulent inflammatory processes in the skin

- Active herpes
- Allergy to peeling components
- Skin integrity disorders
- Pregnancy, lactation
- Thyroid dysfunction
- Diabetes mellitus
- Autoimmune diseases
- Sunburn
- Fungal skin lesions
- Keloid scars
- Couperosis
- Large nevi on the face
- During radiation therapy and chemotherapy
- Less than two weeks after a laser or IPL procedure

There are also modified Jessner peel formulas. For example, resorcinol is replaced by citric or glycolic acid, and ethanol is combined with other alcohols to reduce its concentration.

1.4. Acid peels

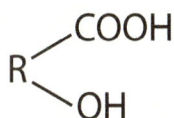

α-hydroxy acids (alpha hydroxy acids; AHAs) are a class of organic compounds with mixed functions, being a carboxylic acid with a hydroxy group located one carbon atom away from the acid group. AHAs are well soluble in highly polar solvents (water, methanol, ethanol, acetone, acetic acid, ethyl acetate), slightly soluble in ethyl ether, and virtually insoluble in nonpolar hydrophobic hydrocarbons.

1.4.1. Mechanism of action

The following AHAs are used in cosmetic dermatology and skincare: glycolic, lactic, mandelic, malic, tartaric, and citric acid. All these substances are found in fruits, so they became known as **fruit acids**. They act by changing the pH gradient through the *stratum corneum*, the importance of which for the work of enzymes was already mentioned (see Part II, section 2.2). Accordingly, the pH change is the "leverage" of acid peels on the skin. However, in addition to enzyme failure, a change in pH gradient affects the structures that maintain the integrity of the *stratum corneum*:

■ Intercellular lipid layers that "glue" corneocytes
■ Corneodesmosomes that form protein bridges between neighboring corneocytes

These structures contain molecules with charged groups, between which there are electrostatic interactions. As the pH of the environment changes, these interactions weaken, which means that the *stratum corneum* becomes looser and less strong. Thus, the change in pH gradient through the *stratum corneum* "hits" three key points that control the barrier formation and ensure its integrity (**Fig. III-1-6**):

1. Enzymes
2. Intercellular lipid layers
3. Corneodesmosomes

The more the pH gradient is changed and the longer this condition lasts, the stronger the desquamation is. The strength of an acid peel, therefore, depends on the pH of the preparation and the exposure time. The acids concentration is not important here: for example, a preparation with a concentration of AHA up to 70% and a pH of 5.5 does

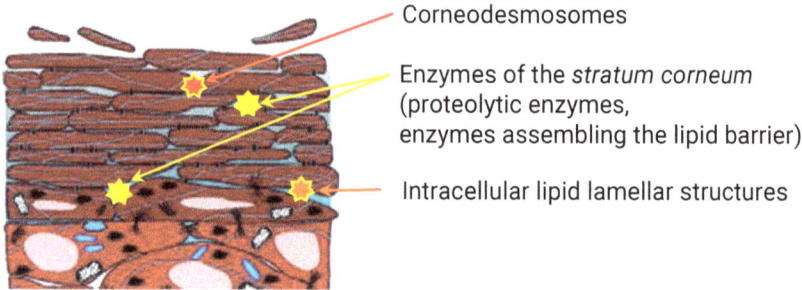

Corneodesmosomes

Enzymes of the *stratum corneum* (proteolytic enzymes, enzymes assembling the lipid barrier)

Intracellular lipid lamellar structures

Figure III-1-6. Targets for acid peels

not exfoliate. On the contrary, a product with 30% AHA and a pH of 1.5 causes noticeable scaling.

The burning sensation that appears some time after applying acid peel indicates that the acidification has gone beyond the *stratum corneum*. Nerve endings, distributed in the skin with high density, communicate with all skin cells — mast cells, endothelial cells, keratinocytes, Langerhans cells, and fibroblasts. In response to an external stimulus (e.g., a decrease in pH of the intercellular space), nerve endings release neuropeptides, such as substance P (SP) or calcitonin gene-related peptide (CGRP), acting on neighboring cells (**Fig. III-1-7**). In turn, the cells release histamine and proinflammatory cytokines, which activate sensory nerve endings and trigger a signal transmission to the brain — this is the signal we perceive as burning.

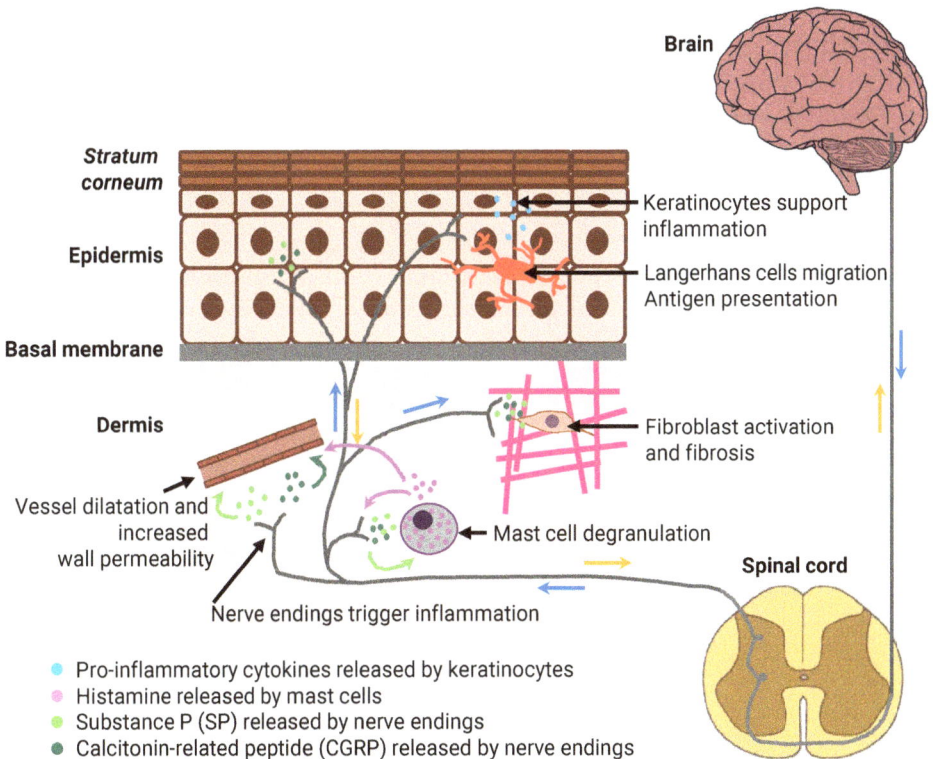

Brain

Stratum corneum

Epidermis

Basal membrane

Keratinocytes support inflammation

Langerhans cells migration Antigen presentation

Dermis

Fibroblast activation and fibrosis

Vessel dilatation and increased wall permeability

Mast cell degranulation

Spinal cord

Nerve endings trigger inflammation

- Pro-inflammatory cytokines released by keratinocytes
- Histamine released by mast cells
- Substance P (SP) released by nerve endings
- Calcitonin-related peptide (CGRP) released by nerve endings

Figure III-1-7. Neurogenic inflammation in the skin

Histamine dilates blood vessels and provides blood flow to the problem area to dissolve and expel irritants as quickly as possible (Choi J.E., Di Nardo A., 2018). If the acid action is not stopped, an inflammatory reaction (so-called **neurogenic inflammation**) is triggered in the epidermis.

Whether it is necessary to provoke an inflammatory reaction in this way is a matter of debate because the main goal of peeling — desquamation — can be achieved without it. Some practitioners believe that inflammation is appropriate if, in addition to exfoliation, we want to activate remodeling processes in the dermal layer. This activation is indirect and is triggered by mediators released by epidermal cells. Other practitioners prefer more effective and comfortable dermal remodeling using injection and physical techniques, and chemical peeling is performed for epidermal exfoliation.

The neutralizer is an alkaline solution in which sodium bicarbonate is usually the main active ingredient and can be used at any time to stop the effects of acid peels. Additionally, it can include moisturizing and softening agents such as β-glucan, plant extracts, and free amino acids.

The clinical effects of hydroxy acids on the skin can be divided into two groups:

1. **Nonspecific effects** typical of all AHAs are determined by the pH of the finished product and consist of accelerating desquamation and renewal of the epidermal cell composition, which is clinically expressed in the characteristic skin scaling.
2. **Specific effects** are related to the chemical characteristics and concentration of a particular AHA and are based on the effect on a specific target in the skin.

The severity of these effects depends on the peel's prescription features and the skin's initial condition.

1.4.2. Fruit acids (α-hydroxy acids)

Glycolic acid

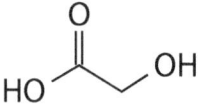

Glycolic acid (2-hydroxyethanoic acid) is the simplest hydroxy acid. It is found in sugarcane and green grapes.

Glycolic acid has the smallest molecular weight among all AHAs and therefore penetrates the epidermal barrier faster than others. It is most often used in acid peels because it can achieve effective exfoliation. The concentration of glycolic acid in peels can be up to 70%. As we have already mentioned, it is not the concentration that determines the strength of exfoliation but the pH, which can be adjusted to the desired level at any acid concentration.

Glycolic acid has other interesting properties, but they appear at low concentrations (about 1–2%). Thus, treatment with a 2% glycolic acid solution increases skin resistance to ultraviolet (UV) radiation and can be considered prevention of photoaging. The fine mechanisms of this effect are under investigation, but it is already known that in the skin pretreated in this way, UV-induced processes develop less intensively. Thus, UV exposure inhibits the expression of aquaporin-3 (a transmembrane protein that forms the channel for the transport of water and osmolytes into the cell and is involved in the regulation of water balance in the living skin layers). It also increases the activity of matrix metalloproteinases (MMPs) that degrade collagen, resulting in clinical manifestations of photoaging, such as skin dehydration and early wrinkles. These processes are less pronounced in the skin treated with glycolic acid preparations. In addition, in the skin treated with 2% glycolic acid, the selection of reactive oxygen species (ROS) and pro-inflammatory mediators after UV radiation is reduced, so erythema is less pronounced than in the untreated area (Hung S.J. et al., 2017; Tang S. G., Yang J.-H., 2018).

Lactic acid

H_3C ... O ... OH ... OH

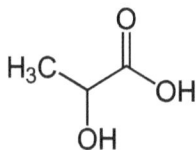

Lactic acid (α-oxypropionic, 2-hydroxypropanoic acid) is a single-base carboxylic acid with three carbon atoms containing a hydroxyl group. Salts and esters of lactic acid are called lactates. Lactic acid is formed by the lactic fermentation of sugars and plays an important role in metabolism.

Lactic (2-hydroxypropanoic) acid was first isolated in 1780. L-lactic acid is produced by the *Lactobacillus* bacteria and is responsible for the smell of fermented milk. D-lactic acid, also called sarcolactic acid, is produced by anaerobic muscle contraction. In nature, D-lactic acid is found in apples, ergot, foxglove, opium, tomatoes, blueberries, passionflower, maple syrup, and grapes.

It is a component of the NMF and has a pronounced moisturizing and mild exfoliating effect on the skin, so it is often used in moisturizing care products. It is included in chemical peels to reduce irritation and soften their effect on the skin (for example, Jessner peel, see Part III, section 1.4).

It is especially recommended for the care of infants and dry skin of the elderly — in these life periods, there is a physiological deficiency of NMF, and the application of a cream in which lactic acid is combined with ceramides and squalene is a great help and provides prolonged hydration.

Citric acid

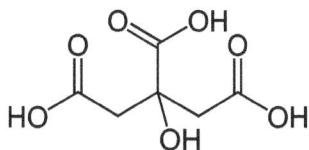

Citric acid is a tribasic carboxylic acid. It is found in various fruits, citrus fruits in particular (up to about 5% in fruits and up to 9% in juice). Citric acid is involved in the tricarboxylic acid cycle — the main process of cell respiration — so in some appreciable concentrations, it is found in all animals and plants.

Citric acid has the highest molecular weight of all the aforementioned AHAs. In skincare products, it is more often used as a pH regulator. Still, in addition to its technical function, citric acid exhibits biological properties — it lightens the skin (especially in the presence of tartaric acid) and has an antioxidant and bactericidal effect.

Mandelic acid

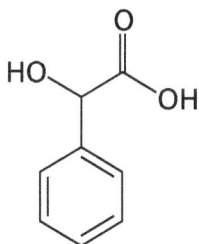

Mandelic acid is the first representative of aromatic hydroxy acids with an aliphatic chain. It is a colorless crystalline solid substance, slightly soluble in water, while dissolving well in polar organic solvents, such as alcohols and diethyl ether. Mandelic acid is obtained by hydrolysis of bitter almond extract.

Mandelic acid is quite mild on the skin. Therefore, it is used in combination with other AHAs in peels and in moisturizing products for regular skincare (Yevglevskis M. et al., 2014).

Tartaric acid

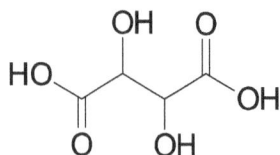

Tartaric acid is a dibasic oxyacid. It is widely distributed in the plant world as free isomers and acidic salts. Its primary source are mature grapes. The substance is released during the fermentation of berry juice, forming hard-to-dissolve potassium salts called tartrate. The food additive is registered under code E334 and is obtained from secondary wine processing products (yeast, chalky sediment, tartaric lime).

When applied to the skin, tartaric acid has an exfoliating, whitening, moisturizing, and antioxidant effect. It is found in peels and in cosmetic products for skin with uneven pigmentation and signs of photoaging.

Malic acid

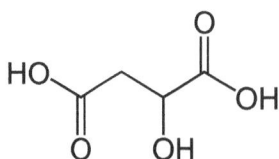

Malic acid is a dibasic keto acid, first isolated from unripe apples in 1785. It is an intermediate product of the tricarboxylic acid and glyoxylate cycles. It is found in many fruits, especially apples, grapes, and rowanberries.

Malic acid has antioxidant, cleansing, moisturizing, anti-inflammatory, and slightly astringent properties. In addition to exfoliating at the *stratum corneum* level, it activates metabolic processes in living cells. It is found in light acid peels. Some studies show a positive effect of malic acid on the skin in atopic dermatitis (Tang S.-C., Yang J. H., 2018; Lee B. et al., 2019).

Pyruvic acid

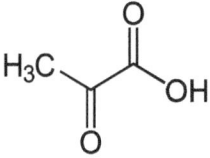

Pyruvic acid is an α-keto analog of lactic acid formed in cells during the pyrolysis of tartaric acid. It plays an important role in cell metabolism, acting as a "crossroads" of many metabolic pathways, particularly in glucose metabolism.

When used topically, pyruvic acid has keratolytic, bactericidal, and sebostatic properties. Due to its low pH value and small size, pyruvic acid passes well through the *stratum corneum*. It can be used to treat dermatological problems such as acne, superficial scars, photodamage, and pigmentation disorders.

A peel in which pyruvic acid is the main active ingredient is called a **Red Peel**. Red Peel is designed for superficial and medium-depth peeling, and contains no more than 50% pyruvic acid in its composition. Upon application, pyruvic acid causes a strong burning sensation, and a little later, erythema develops along with intense scaling (up to crusting). Antioxidant and moisturizing components are added to the formulations to reduce discomfort and the aforementioned consequences, so modern preparations are milder than similar concentrations of pure pyruvic acid solutions.

A comparison of pyruvic acid peels (50%) and salicylic acid peels (30%) in the treatment of mild to moderate acne showed no differences in therapeutic and adverse effects (Jaffary F. et al., 2016). But a comparison of pyruvic acid peeling (50%) and peeling with a combination of glycolic and salicylic acids showed that their therapeutic effectiveness in treating acne is comparable. However, the combined peeling is milder in terms of procedure tolerability and unwanted reactions such as burning sensation, erythema, and edema (Zdrada J. et al., 2020).

1.4.3. Indications, contraindications, and safety precautions for the use of AHA-containing cosmetic products

The main indications for using AHA-containing skincare products are summarized in **Table III-1-2**.

Table III-1-2. Indications for cosmetic products with AHAs

SKIN CONDITION	MECHANISM OF ACTION AND CLINICAL EFFECTS
Dry skin	The total moisture content of the *stratum corneum* is increased by strengthening its water-holding and water-regulating systems: • removal of old corneocytes from the surface promotes the faster renewal of the cellular composition and strengthening of the barrier function of the epidermis (TEWL is reduced, NMF is increased); • stimulation of restoration of intercellular lipid layers of the *stratum corneum*
Oily skin prone to blackheads	• Reducing the cohesion of corneocytes facilitates the clearing of blocked sebaceous gland ducts • Exfoliation opens the sebaceous ducts and makes sebaceous glands accessible to biologically active components that reduce fat formation, normalize lipid metabolism, have a bactericidal effect, etc. • Reducing the likelihood of scarring in acne disease • Prevention and treatment of hyperpigmentation that can occur with acne disease
Fading skin	• Renewing the epidermal cellular composition by exfoliating and proliferating basal keratinocytes • Facilitating penetration into the deeper layers of the skin of other active ingredients in the formulation • Moisturizing effect • Smoothing the skin by increasing its hydration and stimulating the synthesis of collagen and glycosaminoglycans
Pigmented skin	• Facilitating the penetration of bleaching agents into the skin • Direct whitening effect of some AHAs (e.g., tartaric and citric acids)

Without exception, patients with thin, non-greasy skin and minimal pigmentation are more sensitive to AHA than patients with oily and pigmented skin. General advice for those considering the AHA use: start with low concentrations and gradually move up to higher ones, carefully observing the tolerance of the product. Sometimes irritation does not occur immediately but after prolonged use. In this case, you should stop using it, at least temporarily.

Contraindications for AHA formulations:
- Individual intolerance
- Skin hypersensitivity
- Skin injury
- Herpetic lesions
- Telangiectasia
- Prolonged sun exposure

Certain **basic safety precautions** should be followed when using topical AHA-containing products:

1. Always protect your skin before going outdoors. Use sunscreen with a sun protection factor (SPF) of at least 15 (in warm weather, at least 30). Wear a hat and clothing that covers the treated areas of your skin.
2. Use preparations that contain all the necessary information:
   - complete list of ingredients
   - AHA concentration
   - pH value
   - manufacturer's or distributor's name and address

   The first three items are mandatory; the fourth is optional.
3. Before using the product, you should do a control test — apply a small amount of the substance on the back of your hand and watch the reaction overnight.
4. Discontinue use immediately if signs of an adverse reaction appear. These signs include burning, redness, itching, tingling, pain, bleeding, or increased sensitivity to sunlight.

   Adhering to these measures is not difficult, and they can protect against serious problems arising from a seemingly innocuous and promising cosmetic product.

After acid peeling, the skin becomes clearer and brighter. The overall clinical result is due to the diverse biological action of AHAs. In the epidermis, AHAs activate cell renewal, which reduces the *stratum corneum*'s thickness and increases its hydration, and through exfoliation reduces the amount of melanin in the epidermis and lightens the skin. The anti-inflammatory activity of AHAs is due to their antioxidant properties and ability to influence inflammatory mediators' release. With long-term use of skincare products with AHAs, a slight lifting effect may be observed owing to the improved dermal matrix quality. However, this effect is related to an indirect effect on fibroblasts through cytokines that are released by epidermal cells in response to AHAs.

1.4.4. Polyhydroxy acids

How can the beneficial properties of AHAs be attained without the burning risk? Many pharmaceutical and cosmetic companies are working in this direction. One option is using polyhydroxy acids (PHAs) — they are better tolerated by the skin and moisturize it better than glycolic acid, which is traditionally used as a peeling agent. Several PHAs were selected based on the results obtained in research studies.

Gluconic acid and gluconolactone

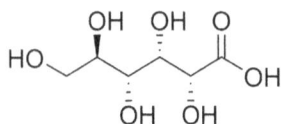

Gluconic acid is an organic acid of the aldonic acid group with $C_6H_{12}O_7$ chemical formula. It is formed by the oxidation of the aldehyde group of glucose. The phosphorylated form of gluconic acid is an important intermediate product of carbohydrate metabolism in living cells. The compound activates metabolism in the body, increases muscle performance, and has other beneficial effects on the body.

Gluconic acid and its derivative, gluconolactone, are used in skin-care. Both compounds are characterized by good moisturizing and mild keratolytic action, an optimal combination for the care of very dry and sensitive skin. They also have antioxidant properties that are useful for seriously compromised skin barrier. Ichthyosis patients have insufficient protease activity of the *stratum corneum*, which results in impaired desquamation.

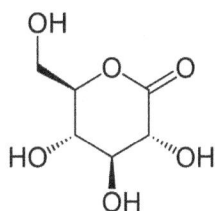

Gluconolactone is a lactone (cyclic ester) of D-gluconic acid obtained by bacterial fermentation of pure glucose to form gluconic acid and subsequent solution evaporation. It is a white crystalline powder with a faint characteristic odor. It is soluble in water and glycerine and insoluble in ethyl alcohol and vegetable oil.

PHAs do not increase the skin's sensitivity to sunlight and can be used as a part of a treatment protocol that includes retinoids and other cosmetic products. Since the molecules of these substances are larger than those of AHAs, they penetrate much more slowly, allowing the substance to accumulate within the *stratum corneum*. This is a big advantage in this case because the task of the PHAs is to act on the *stratum corneum*, not on living cells.

Gluconolactone is gentler than gluconic acid, which is why it is especially recommended for severe pathologies such as ichthyosis. The acid (carboxyl) group in gluconolactone is "masked" and contact with the skin does not cause burning. During hydrolysis, the ring "unfolds" and the lactone turns into the α-form, gluconic acid, a substance natural to cells. By acidifying the *stratum corneum*, gluconolactone activates proteases that break down corneodesmosomes, facilitating corneocyte desquamation.

Lactobionic acid

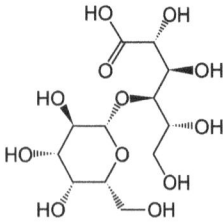

Lactobionic acid is a 4-O-β-D-galacto-pyranosyl-D-gluconic acid consisting of gluconic acid and galactose. It may be formed during the oxidation of the disaccharide lactose. It forms salts with metals such as calcium, potassium, sodium, and zinc.

Lactobionic acid is a hybrid consisting of galactose sugar and gluconic acid (according to the classification, it belongs to the class of bionic polyhydroxy acids). A molecule of lactobionic acid has eight hydroxyl groups, meaning it can "bind" eight water molecules to itself by ionic bonds (for comparison: gluconolactone has four hydroxyl groups, and lactic and glycolic acids have one each). So, lactobionic acid is an excellent moisturizer, acting in a "similar way" to the NMF components. Moreover, its water-absorbing and water-holding properties are superior to those of most hygroscopic compounds traditionally used in topical preparations (Tasić-Kostov M. et al., 2019).

The safety of lactobionic acid is proven, due to which it is used (usually in salt form) in the food industry and pharmacy. Thus, calcium lactobionate is used as a food stabilizer. Potassium lactobionate is added to special solutions designed for the osmotic stabilization of cells and tissues. The mineral salts of lactobionate are used as mineral food additives. The antibiotic erythromycin is used in salt form (erythromycin lactobionate) when administered intravenously. Experiments have also revealed the positive effects of lactobionic acid on the dermal matrix. It is assumed that it inhibits matrix metalloproteinases, "slowing down" the destruction of collagen and elastin. After long-term use of preparations with lactobionic acid, the biomechanical properties of the skin, including elasticity and tensile strength, improve.

All these qualities make lactobionic acid a valuable ingredient in topical preparations designed for:

- deep and long-lasting hydration (dry and very dry skin, skin with damaged *stratum corneum*, photodamaged skin)
- restorative care after aesthetic procedures (such as microdermabrasion, chemical peeling, non-ablative phototherapy, mesotherapy)

Thanks to their dermatological mildness, PHAs can be used to care for skin with a weak barrier and increased sensitivity. PHAs are also useful for the care of photodamaged skin the barrier properties of which have been damaged by high doses of UV radiation. Delicately acting at the level of the *stratum corneum*, the PHAs help to smooth out the skin microrelief, restore hydration, and even out skin tone.

1.5. Retinol peels

Retinol peels are fundamentally different from keratolytic, acidic, and enzymatic peels in that they stimulate rather than damage their targets. This is the only category of chemical peels for which the targets are living cells, more precisely, their nuclei that have receptors for *trans*-retinoic acid. Retinoids are substances that regulate the expression of a variety of genes, and the genes are the levers that trigger first the cellular and then the tissue response to retinoid exposure.

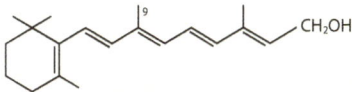

Retinol (true vitamin A) is a oil-soluble vitamin, an antioxidant, and refers to organic alcohols (–OH). In the form of alcohol, it is found only in animal products. In plant foods, it is present in the form of β-carotene (precursor of vitamin A). In cells, it is converted to the active form — retinoic acid.

1.5.1. Mechanism of action

The biologically active form is not retinol itself, but its derivative — *trans*-retinoic acid (*trans*-RA, better known among practitioners as tretinoin), which is formed in the cells themselves in two steps: first, retinol is oxidized to retinal, which is in turn, is oxidized to *trans*-RA. Another retinol derivative, 9-*cis*-RA, which also exhibits physiological activity, is formed from *trans*-RA (**Fig. III-1-8**). It is also possible to transform retinol to inactive metabolites (**Fig. III-1-9**).

Cells are very sensitive to retinol concentration, and even minor deviation from the norm affects their vital functions. The mechanism of cellular regulation of retinoid metabolism is a complex and well-established system. It includes many enzymes and binding proteins that ensure retinoid capture, metabolism, deposition, and transport inside the cell.

After penetrating the plasma membrane inside the cell, retinoids are metabolized to active derivatives and bind to special proteins. In this form, they are delivered to the nucleus, where they are recognized by retinoid receptors (**Fig. III-1-10**). The activated receptor,

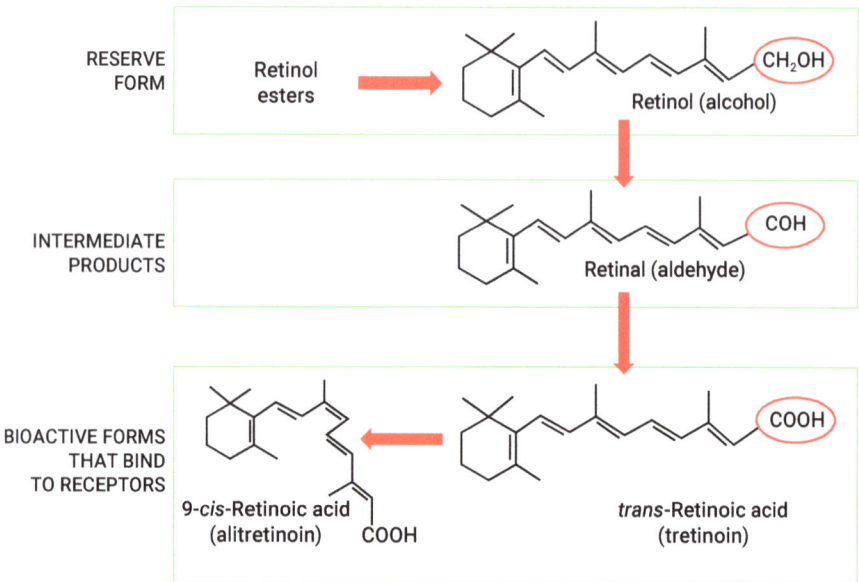

Figure III-1-8. Biotransformation of vitamin A in the cell

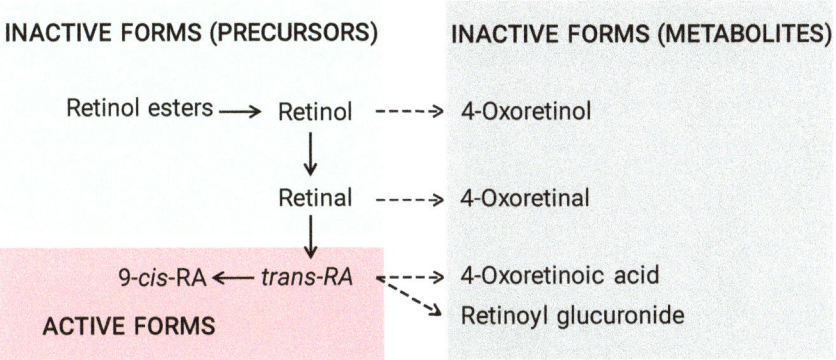

INACTIVE FORMS (PRECURSORS)	INACTIVE FORMS (METABOLITES)
Retinol esters ⟶ Retinol ----→	4-Oxoretinol
Retinal ----→	4-Oxoretinal
9-*cis*-RA ⟵ *trans*-RA ←---→	4-Oxoretinoic acid
ACTIVE FORMS	Retinoyl glucuronide

Figure III-1-9. Intracellular (endogenous) retinoids: precursors represent the stock of retinol in the cell, and metabolites result from inactivation and utilization of retinoids by the cell

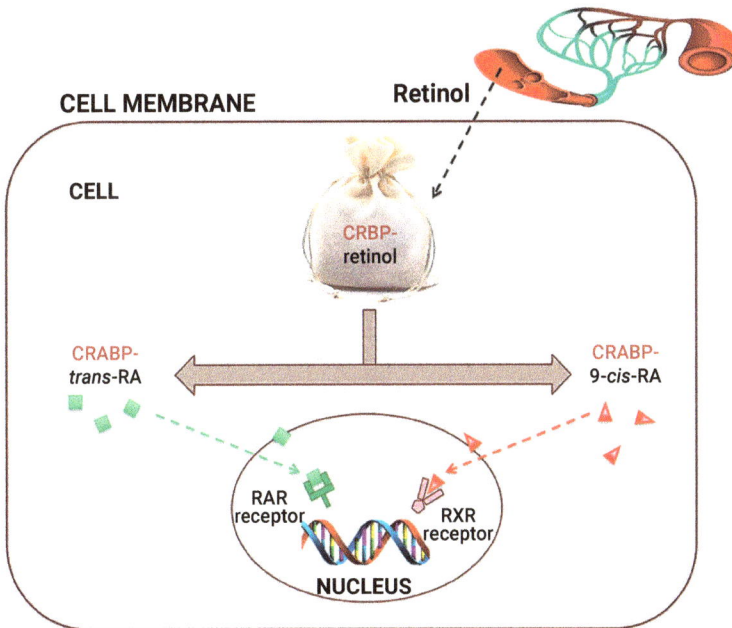

Figure III-1-10. Regulation of retinol levels in the cell

Intracellular retinoid-binding proteins:
- CRBP (cellular retinol-binding protein) — retinol deposition in the cell
- CRABP (cellular retinoic acid-binding protein) — retinoic acid delivery to the nucleus

Each class of intracellular retinoid-binding proteins has types 1 and 2.

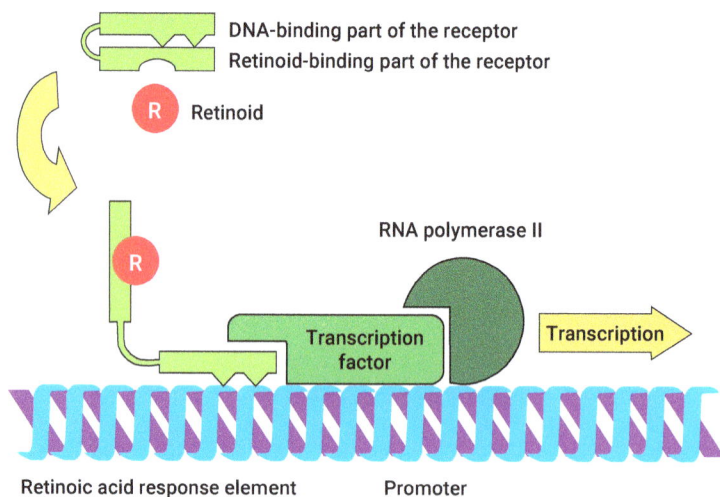

Figure III-1-11. Activation of target gene expression by retinoic receptors

Retinoid receptors:
• RARs (retinoic acid receptors)
• RXRs (retinoid X receptors)
Each receptor family has three receptor isoforms (α, β, γ).

in turn, binds to a short deoxyribonucleic acid (DNA) sequence near the promoter of the target gene and stabilizes the transcription factor (**Fig. III-1-11**). The role of the transcription factor is to ensure that the ribonucleic acid (RNA) polymerase II enzyme binds to the promoter and triggers transcription.

The above scheme is greatly simplified. In reality, the process is more complicated. Retinoic acid receptors are divided into two groups: RARs (retinoic acid receptors) and RXRs (retinoid X receptors), each with three isoforms (α, β, γ). Thus, the retinoic acid receptor system includes six types of receptors.

As for intracellular retinoid-binding proteins, there are two major classes: cellular retinol-binding proteins (CRBPs) and cellular retinoic acid-binding proteins (CRABPs). Each protein class has subclasses I and II. These highly specific proteins show great affinity to their ligands (retinol and retinoic acid, respectively). The exact function of these proteins is still unclear. It is assumed that CRBPs play an important role in retinoid metabolism and deposit retinol in the cell. As for CRABPs,

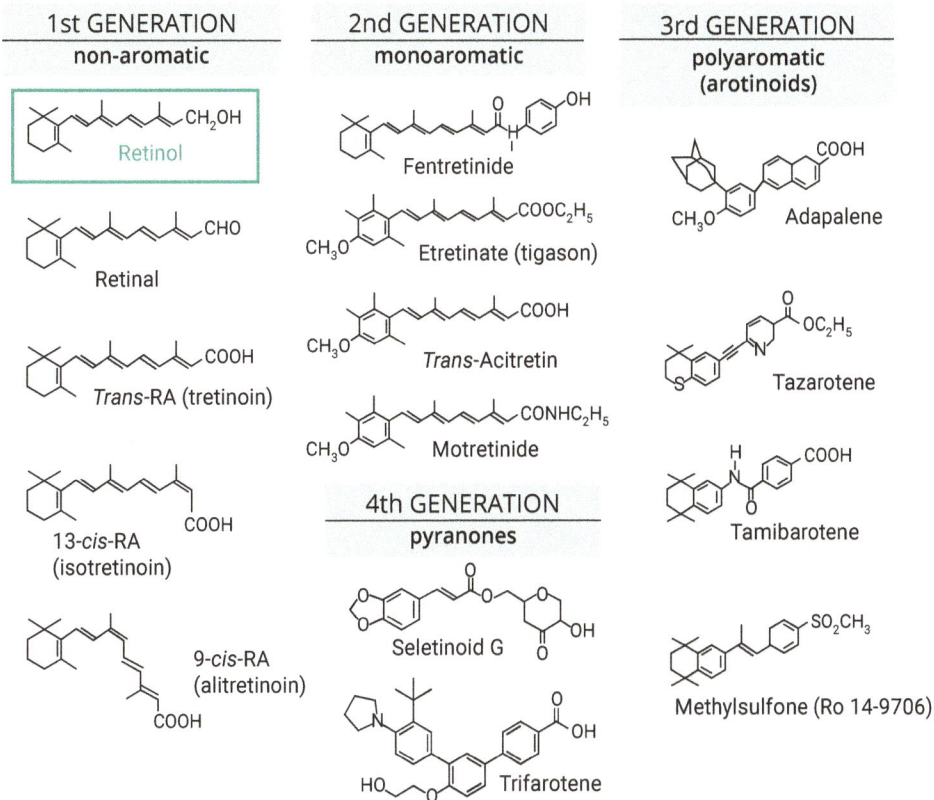

Figure III-1-12. Retinoids in clinical practice

they presumably perform transport functions and deliver the *trans*-RA to the nucleus, where it binds to its receptor.

Over time, scientists have found substances that have similar effects to vitamin A. Synthetic and natural compounds with retinol-like mechanism of action began to be called retinoids and used to treat various diseases, including skin disorders (Krężel W. et al., 2019). **Fig. III-1-12** shows examples of retinoids used in clinical practice. The 1st generation retinoids are natural compounds because they are retinol derivatives found in the cells. The other substances are not found in nature and belong to synthetic retinoids. The 4th generation retinoids — selectinoid G and tripharotene — are considered promising candidates for use in dermatology and skincare. Both substances are selective agonists of RAR-γ, the most common receptor type for retinoic acid in the skin.

There are also ingredients of plant origin that can be converted to retinol in the human body or have a retinol-like effect on cells. The first group includes β-carotene. When ingested with food, it is converted into retinol, i.e., a pro-vitamin A. This happens in the intestinal cells because they have the necessary enzyme for this — dioxygenase. When applied topically, β-carotene in the skin remains β-carotene because skin cells do not have this enzyme. β-carotene has no affinity to nuclear retinoid receptors, i.e., it cannot influence the cell's genetic apparatus like retinoids do. But this does not mean that β-carotene and carotenoids are useless in skincare products — they are good antioxidants that help the skin to resist oxidative stress and increase its resistance to UV rays (Stahl W., Sies H., 2012). Still, when applied topically, the clinical effects typical for retinoids will be absent.

The second group includes substances that can bind to nuclear retinoid receptors (Chaudhuri R. K., Bojanowski K., 2014). This binding is much weaker than that of retinoids. While their clinical effects (including adverse reactions) are not as pronounced as those of real retinoids, they act on cells like retinoids. Bacuchiol, derived from psoralea witch hazel seeds, belongs to this group. Today, this substance is popular and can be found in products for the treatment of age-related skin changes and for skin with increased sebum production (Dhaliwal S. et al., 2019).

1.5.2. Cosmetics or medicine?

Several questions need to be addressed separately: How should retinoid-based topical products be classified? Why are some registered as drugs with all the ensuing requirements for sale and prescription, while others are sold uncontrolled and classified as cosmetics?

To begin with, all synthetic retinoids are medicinal substances not approved for cosmetics use.

As for natural retinoids (endogenous derivatives of vitamin A), it all depends on their form:

- biologically active *trans*-RA or 13-*cis*-RA are drugs
- precursors (retinol, retinal, retinol esters) are cosmetic ingredients

Recall that cells store retinol and convert it into the active form as needed, which binds to nuclear receptors. If the cell is "fed" with *trans*-RA, it will no longer be able to self-regulate the number of active molecules it needs, and the cellular response will be forced, fast, and pronounced. If retinol or its esters get into the cell, they are deposited and then gradually activated, so the effect is slow and less prominent. **Cosmetic products are based on an intracrine concept: precursors are applied onto the skin and are transformed into a biologically active form in the skin cells (Fig. III-1-13).** Accordingly, it is correct to say retinol skincare products and retinoid medication (**Fig. III-1-14**).

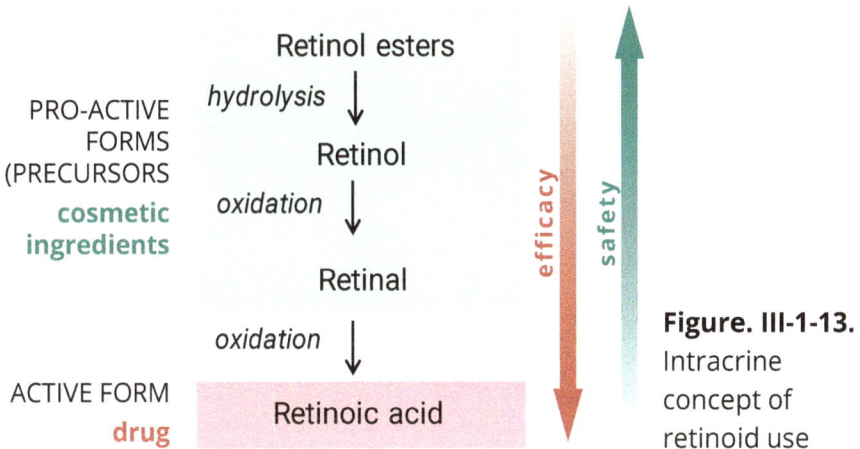

PRO-ACTIVE FORMS (PRECURSORS
cosmetic ingredients

Retinol esters

hydrolysis ↓

Retinol

oxidation ↓

Retinal

oxidation ↓

efficacy   safety

ACTIVE FORM
drug

Retinoic acid

Figure. III-1-13. Intracrine concept of retinoid use

COSMETICS	DRUG
Interaction with nuclear receptors	Interaction with nuclear receptors
NO	**YES**

Inactive forms (precursor or metabolites)
- Retinol esters
- **Retinol (pure vitamin A)**
- Retinal
- Oxoretinoids

Bioactive forms:
- *trans*-RA (tretinoin)
- 9-*cis*-RA (alitretinoin)
- 13-*cis*-RA (isotretinoin)
- Synthetic retinoids

Figure III-1-14. Cosmetics or medicine: the principle of retinoid selection

Table III-1-3. Recommended doses of retinol, retinyl palmitate, and retinyl acetate in cosmetic products (assuming an initial concentration of 1 million IU/g)

RETINOL, %	RETINYL PALMITATE, %	RETINYL ACETATE, %
Day cream 0.5–0.1	Cream/Lotion ..0.1–0.5	Day cream 0.5–5.0
Night cream 0.1–0.2	Shampoo 0.1–0.5	Night cream . 0.5–5.0
Hand cream 0.05	Conditioner 0.1–0.5	Body milk 0.5–2.0
Body milk 0.05–0.1	Nail care	After-sun
After-sun cream 0.1–0.2	products 0.1–0.5	face cream 3.0–5.0
After-sun body milk .. 0.05–0.1		After-sun
Peel cream .... **app. 1%**		body milk 1.0–3.0
(up to 10%)		

Another important issue to consider when designing treatment is the dose of retinoids. The choice of vitamin A and its esters concentrations depends on the cosmetic product's purpose (**Table III-1-3**) and the treatment objectives. Skincare products are used permanently and are intended for the physiological regulation of skin cells to prevent/treat signs of aging and photoaging, and control the activity of sebum production. Peel preparations are designed to stimulate active desquamation and used once. In products for routine care, retinol concentration is usually lower than average. Products for treating symptoms of photodamage have higher concentrations. The highest concentration of retinol (around 1%) is found in products for intensive rejuvenation, which are essentially peel products.

The presence of nuclear receptors and similarities in the molecular mechanisms of activation give scientists reason to put retinol on par with the steroid and thyroid hormones since their action is also mediated through nuclear receptors. Moreover, the nuclear receptors for retinoids, steroids, and thyroids are similar in structure and mechanism of action and can even influence each other's activity. This explains, in particular, the fact that vitamin D (steroid precursor) acts synergistically with vitamin A, stimulating its uptake and metabolism in keratinocytes.

1.5.3. Retinoid effects

The clinical manifestations of retinoids are so diverse that it is hard to believe that one or even a few genes are responsible for all of them. The effects of retinol on the skin have been compared to an iceberg: we only see the tip — the clinical effects that result from changes in the cells deep within the skin (Riahi R.R. et al., 2016). To understand the visible effects of retinol, it is important to remember that it only acts on living cells, with different cell types responding differently, as shown in **Table III-1-4** focusing on its impact on the skin.

Table III-1-4. Effects of retinoids on the skin at different levels

LEVEL	EFFECTS
Clinical	• Visible scaling • Skin lightening • Smoothing wrinkles • Accelerated wound healing • Improved skin firmness and elasticity • Irritation
Histological	• Thinning of the *stratum corneum* • Thickening of the living layers of the epidermis • Changing the structure of the dermis (restoration of the collagen matrix)
Cellular	• Stimulation of basal keratinocyte proliferation • Stimulation of fibroblasts to the synthesis of intercellular matrix components • Suppression of sebocytes' secretory activity
Immunological	• Stimulation of Langerhans cells to present antigens • Induction of keratinocyte expression of intercellular adhesive molecules that play an important role in intercellular communication and development of immune response • Modulation of production of some cytokines, including those involved in inflammatory and immune reactions

Continued on p. 98

LEVEL	EFFECTS
Biochemical	• Regulation of keratinocyte differentiation (in particular, influence on keratin and involucrin expression) • Regulation of the activity of enzymes involved in melanin synthesis • Reduction of keratinocyte production of vascular endothelial growth factor, which affects the development of blood capillaries in the skin • Regulation of lipid and keratin synthesis in sebocytes • Reducing the level and activity of dermal metalloproteinases and connective tissue enzymes that degrade the intercellular matrix
Molecular	• Effect on the level of intracellular retinoic acid binding proteins • Activation of gene expression through nuclear receptors (RARs and RXRs)

Each year, numerous articles on the effects of retinoids (both desirable and undesirable) are published in the scientific and medical literature (Khalil S. et al., 2017). We have compiled what we consider the most interesting facts, paying particular attention to those that have direct implications for dermatology and skincare (**Table III-1-5**).

1.5.4. Features of retinoid use

Retinoids are small, lipophilic molecules. They easily penetrate the *stratum corneum* and the pilosebaceous unit (sebaceous gland associated with the hair follicle). A retinoid concentration gradient is created in the skin, decreasing towards the dermis. In the epidermis, retinoids control keratinization and pigmentation processes. In the dermal layer, they restore the intercellular matrix that is gradually degraded due to aging or UV exposure. The transfollicular pathway makes it possible to obtain an increased retinoid concentration in the hair follicles, which is especially valuable in treating follicular pathologies, including acne.

In intensive treatment preparations, retinol concentration is higher than in products for regular care. Special creamy masks (containing up

Table III-1-5. Main cellular "targets" of retinol in the skin responsible for clinical outcome

TARGET CELL	CELLULAR RESPONSE	HISTOLOGICAL CHANGES	CLINICAL OUTCOME
Keratino-cyte	• Stimulation of division, maturation, and migration	• Updating the cellular composition of the epidermis • Thinning of the *stratum corneum*	• Smoothing of microrelief, reduction of keratosis signs • Reducing the expression of wrinkles • Tone leveling • In case of an excessive dose — dryness of the *stratum corneum*
Sebocyte	• Suppression of sebum production	• Reducing the amount of sebum • Normalization of the sebum composition	• Reducing oily shine
Fibroblast	• Stimulation of synthetic activity	• Changes in the intercellular matrix structure: improvement of the collagen–elastin framework	• Improved skin elasticity and turgor • Smoothing fine lines and wrinkles
Langerhans cell	• Modulation of the antigen-presenting ability • Reduced production of inflammatory mediators in keratinocytes	• Restoration of vascular wall permeability • Reduction of tissue infiltration by immunocytes	• Reduction of erythema • Reduction of local edema

to 10% retinol) are designed for the professional peeling performed by specialists. Retinol colors the product yellow, so it is called a **Yellow Peel**. *Trans*-RA (5–10% tretinoin) can also be used instead of retinol, but the product must be classified as a drug.

In addition to retinol/retinoic acid, other organic acids, such as salicylic acid, may also be present. Phytic, kojic, and azelaic acids, known for their inhibitory effect on melanin synthesis, are commonly found in cosmetic products. Phytic acid, among other things, is a chelator of divalent ions and binds iron ions, thus preventing the development of oxidative stress in the skin. Hydroquinone is added to some formulations to enhance the whitening power of peels. Vitamins as well as anti-inflammatory and soothing additives (e.g., chamomile extract, aloe, allantoin, vitamin C) can be added to the formulation.

1.5.5. Practical aspects of retinol peeling

Indications for retinol peeling:
- Epidermal melasma
- Pigment spots
- Superficial wrinkles
- Seborrhea
- Post-acne

Contraindications:
- Low-sebum dry skin (e.g., age-related dryness, pathological dryness on the background of diseases, improper use of skincare products, unbalanced diet)
- Taking vitamin A in another form to avoid an overdose
- Current or history of liver disease
- Injuries and skin scratches in the treating area
- Acute stage of acne
- Pregnancy, lactation
- Individual intolerance

The peeling procedure is uncomplicated and easily tolerated. The general protocol is outlined on the next page.

After cleansing, a small concentration of AHA or salicylic acid lotion is rubbed into the skin to increase the permeability of the *stratum corneum* and prepare it for the application of the Yellow Peel.

The Yellow Peel is applied in a thin, even layer to the whole face or a separate area, left for some time (from 20 min to 2 h, depending on the skin condition and retinol concentration), and then washed off with a mild cleanser.

After two hours, the application can be repeated, and this can be done several times depending on the treatment objective. For example, in the case of epidermal melasma, it is enough to make 2–3 repeated applications. This provokes a mild scaling with minimal inflammation. To work with wrinkles, photodamaged skin, and acne, 5–6 applications of four-hour duration may be needed. This will result in pronounced scaling and more inflammation, but the renewal effect will also be more pronounced.

After about a day or two, there is a feeling of tightness, and scaling begins on Days 4–5. After about a week, the skin becomes smoother and fresher. It looks noticeably better after just one treatment, but for the effect to be most pronounced and durable, the course must involve at least three treatments at 10–14 day intervals.

In the post-peeling period, the skin should be treated with a special protective, restorative preparation (vaseline or even hydrocortisone ointment is possible) several times a day for 3–5 days until it regains its barrier structures. Attention should also be paid to moisturizing the skin. After about five days, you can start using bleaching products, but only those that do not contain AHA, retinol, or proteolytic enzymes. If the procedure is performed during the sunny season, during and after the course of retinol peeling, it is necessary to use products with high SPF, because the removal of upper layers renders the skin very sensitive to pigmentation.

The question concerning the depth of retinol peels does not have as clear-cut answer as it seems at first glance. Many publications state that retinol peels are "superficial." It is difficult to agree with this perspective because retinol targets the basal keratinocytes, which is the level of activity of a medium-depth peel.

However, unlike all other peeling agents, retinol stimulates living cells rather than destroying specific skin structures. Therefore, the skin tolerates retinol peeling easily — there is no pain (sometimes there is a slight tingling sensation, but it is insignificant), persistent swelling, and erythema. Severe peeling, a consequence of a sharp imbalance between the rate of division of basal keratinocytes and the rate of desquamation, passes fairly quickly. We can thus state that retinol peeling can achieve non-traumatic and complete renewal of the epidermis at all its levels.

Retinol peeling is recommended once or twice a year. The best time for the procedure is in late fall, winter, and early spring. It is a cosmetic procedure and should be performed by a skincare specialist. Nonetheless, sometimes clients perform it independently at home because it is relatively safe.

1.6. General recommendations for the chemical peel procedure

Table III-1-6 summarizes information on the mechanisms of action and clinical effects of different peeling agents. **Table III-1-7** presents

Table III-1-6. Mechanisms of action and clinical effects of different peeling agents

MECHANISM OF ACTION	MOLECULAR LEVEL	CELLULAR LEVEL	HISTOLOGICAL LEVEL	CLINICAL OUTCOME
Salicylic acid				
Keratolytic, denaturing and destroying protein structures	Breaks intra- and intermolecular protein disulfide bonds	• Weakens cohesion of corneocytes • Reduces the production of inflammatory mediators	• Loosens the *stratum corneum* • Antiseptic • Reduces the synthetic activity of sebocytes	• Exfoliation of the *stratum corneum* • Alignment of microrelief • Lightening and smoothing of skin tone • Reduced sebum production • Reducing inflammation

Continued on p. 103

MECHANISM OF ACTION	MOLECULAR LEVEL	CELLULAR LEVEL	HISTOLOGICAL LEVEL	CLINICAL OUTCOME
AHAs, PHAs				
Changes in the pH of the intercellular medium (acidification) of the *stratum corneum* and the living layers of the epidermis	Change the activity of the *stratum corneum* enzymes, influence on electrostatic interactions of corneodesmosomes	• Increase mitotic activity of basal keratinocytes • Increase the number of lamellar bodies in granular keratinocytes	• Accelerate renewal of the epidermal cellular composition • Thin the *stratum corneum* • Strengthen the barrier function of the *stratum corneum*	• Exfoliation of the *stratum corneum* • Smoothing of microrelief • Lightening and smoothing of skin tone
Proteolytic enzymes				
Weaken the cohesion of corneocytes	Selectively destroy corneodesmosomes as well as protein–lipid contaminants on the skin surface	No effect on epidermal living cells	Stimulate renewal of the epidermis cellular composition by accelerating desquamation	• Skin cleansing • Exfoliation of the *stratum corneum* • Smoothing of microrelief
Retinol and its derivatives				
Control the proliferation of all living cells; rapidly dividing cells are the most sensitive to retinol	Affect the genetic apparatus of living cells through specific nuclear receptors	Regulate the activity of many genes of all skin cell types, incl.: • Keratinocyte genes responsible for cell division, maturation, and migration • Sebocyte genes responsible for sebum production	• Accelerate the processes of cellular renewal of the epidermis • Suppress the activity of sebum production	• Skin exfoliation • Smoothing of microrelief • Normalization of fat separation

Table III-1-7. Classification of chemical peels according to the depth of damage

PEELING TYPE	DEPTH OF DAMAGE	CHEMICAL AGENTS	CLINICAL INDICATIONS	RECOVERY TIME
Exfoliation (very superficial)	*Stratum corneum*	• Proteolytic enzymes • AHAs (10–20%), pH 3.5–4.5	Uneven pigmentation, slight signs of photoaging, fine surface wrinkles, dull complexion	Quick recovery, scaling is almost imperceptible
Surface	*Stratum corneum*, granular layer	• AHAs (20–30%), pH 2.5–3.5 • Jessner solution • Resorcinol (20–30%) • TCA (10%)	Uneven pigmentation, melasma, minor signs of photoaging, fine surface wrinkles	Quick recovery, scaling is almost invisible
Surface/ Medium-depth	*Stratum corneum*, granular layer, spiky layer	• Glycolic acid (50–70%), pH 2.0–3.0 • Salicylic acid • Jessner solution (longer exposure) • Resorcinol (30–50%) • TCA (10–30%)	Hyperpigmentation, melasma, acne, moderate photoaging, wrinkles	Recovery within 1–2 days, more pronounced scaling
Medium-depth/ Deep	All the way down to the basal layer	• Glycolic acid (70%), pH < 1.0 • TCA (up to 50%)	Moderate photoaging, deep wrinkles	Healing usually takes about 7 days, during which there is redness, some swelling, and noticeable scaling

the classification of chemical peels according to the depth of damage (except for retinol, which acts through stimulation of basal keratinocytes rather than destruction).

Protocols for chemical peeling with different compositions differ in detail, but there are common points to remember.

Skin exfoliation with AHAs in low concentrations, scrubs, and enzyme compositions can be performed without prior preparation: in fact, they are used in the preparatory stage of the peeling procedure itself (see Part I, section 2.5) or during the pre-peeling preparation phase, which usually starts 1–2 weeks before the procedure.

Proper skin preparation and subsequent restorative care are essential. Both before and after the peeling procedure, sun exposure should be avoided.

The main aims of pre-peeling treatment:
- Strengthen the skin's reparative potential
- Weaken the barrier properties of the *stratum corneum*
- Even out the microrelief so that the peeling agents penetrate the skin more evenly during the session
- Reduce melanocyte activity to avoid the risk of post-inflammatory pigmentation
- Extinguish inflammation (if there is any)

Preparations and ingredients used for pre-peeling treatment:
- Preparations with AHA up to 20% and pH not lower than 3.0, preparations with retinol of about 0.02% — to weaken the barrier properties of the skin and thus reduce the exposure time and concentration of the peeling agents
- Calcium ion chelators (e.g., phytic acid and EDTA) to reduce corneocytes cohesion
- Depigmenting agents to control the formation of melanin in the skin
- Antioxidant and anti-inflammatory agents

Before applying the peel product, the skin needs to be thoroughly cleaned. The choice of cleansing solution is important because grease and dirt must be removed without irritating and damaging the skin (see Part I, chapter 2).

Unpleasant sensations (pain, burning, tingling) may occur after applying the peel. If they become too strong, the peel should be immediately removed or neutralized (in the case of acid peels). During keratolytic peeling, the depth of penetration is controlled by the frost.

After removing the peel, a soothing and anti-inflammatory cream should be applied to the skin, completing the procedure with a protective cream with UV filters. Usually, it is a cream with occlusive properties — it is necessary to prevent water evaporation, which increases sharply after the peel preparation is applied to the *stratum corneum*. The more severe the damage, the more occlusive the product must be (see Part III, chaper 6 and Part IV, section 1.1).

As the barrier is rebuilt, the post-peeling care changes to include "lighter" moisturizers and emollients. Be sure to use products with UV filters for sun protection and avoid sun exposure if possible.

Basic safety rules:
- Clean the skin thoroughly, but do not allow irritation
- Under-exfoliating is better than over-exfoliating
- For acid peel, carefully neutralize (if necessary) or wash off at the end of the exposure time
- Make sure to apply a protective cream at the end of the procedure

In modern cosmetic dermatology and skincare, chemical peels are increasingly seen as an effective way to treat changes that primarily affect the epidermis. Therefore, superficial light peels are preferred. Structural changes at the level of the dermal layer are treated by injections or physical methods, which due to their minimally invasive nature do not cause severe damage to the skin's barrier structures. Because of this division of "areas of responsibility," chemical peels are successfully combined with other methods of aesthetic medicine, not trying to impose more than they actually can do.

Chapter 2
Concentrates of biologically active ingredients

Using products containing high concentrations of active ingredients is another option for intensive treatment of healthy skin besides peels. Many of these products (just like peels) are multifunctional and allow several aesthetic problems to be solved simultaneously. They are often applied under the mask, creating an occlusion film and ensuring even more active penetration of ingredients through the *stratum corneum* already prepared by cleansing. In some cases, they can also be applied after peeling.

All ingredients discussed in the following sections can also be used in home care products but are usually found in lower concentrations.

2.1. Peptide regulators

The appearance of peptides in the cosmetic market made much noise — some called them a new milestone in cosmetic dermatology and skincare, others treated them with suspicion as just another advertisement. However, even their relatively short use has shown that peptides do not justify the hopes placed on them, although they may surprise us in the future. Even now, a separate niche in anti-aging medicine is occupied by so-called remodeling peptides, which start synthesizing extracellular matrix components. These myorelaxant peptides are considered an alternative to botulinum toxin, neurotransmitter peptides, and many compounds that improve microcirculation. In addition, new substances appear every year, their range of possibilities is expanding, production is becoming cheaper, and the availability of peptides in cosmetic products is increasing.

There is no doubt that peptide skincare products are a trend that will take the lead in aesthetic medicine for many years to come. Let's remember what peptides are and see what new products the cosmetic market offers today.

2.1.1. Basic properties

Peptides are a group of substances with molecules comprising amino acids linked together by peptide bonds. In other words, they are proteins in their chemical structure, but nowadays, they are divided into separate groups. Thus, **proteins** are those amino acid chains that consist of hundreds or more amino acids (for example, a collagen molecule includes about 500 amino acids), while **peptides** are short-chain structures containing only a few (up to tens) amino acid residues (**Fig. III-2-1**).

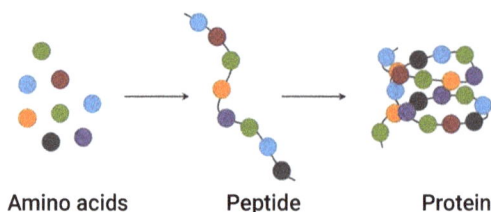

Figure III-2-1. Peptides and proteins

Although there are only 20 amino acids in our body, their sequence in the peptide chain can give rise to countless combinations. Since the sequence of amino acids determines the biological functions of peptides, the potential range of their uses is almost unlimited.

Peptides are particularly valuable for their ability to regulate various aspects of cellular activity. For example, most peptides are signaling molecules: by binding to cell receptors (in the "key-lock" manner), they can "switch" cell functions, triggering or blocking specific processes, such as the synthesis of key proteins of the extracellular matrix, keratinization, or melanogenesis (**Fig. III-2-2**). Since intercellular signaling systems were formed at the earliest stages of evolution, the "orders" encoded in peptides are universal. Human cells can be influenced by peptides from various animals and even plants. In addition, peptides can bind to individual proteins, thus blocking or stimulating their function.

In cosmetic chemistry, it is customary to indicate the number of amino acids that make up a peptide in its very name. For example,

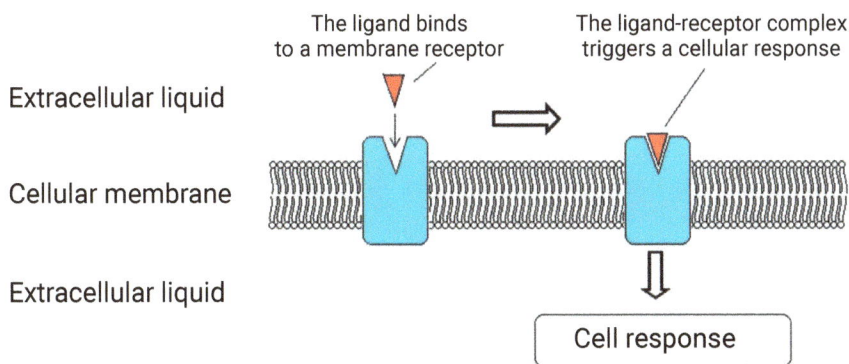

Figure III-2-2. The peptide interacts with the receptor on the cell membrane in the "key–lock" manner

a peptide consisting of two amino acids is called a dipeptide, those which contain three amino acids are called a tripeptide, etc. The most interesting prospects concern using peptides containing 2 to 10 amino acids. The small size of such peptides helps them move easily in the intercellular space and penetrate the skin. The classic rule of 500 Da says that the skin barrier limits the penetration of substances with a larger molecular weight. Since the mass of one amino acid is, on average, 100 Da, small peptides can pass through the *stratum corneum* without additional help (Bos J.D., Meinardi M.M., 2000). However, it should be noted that many peptides are water-soluble compounds, so they are "sewn" a lipophilic "tail" (most often palmitic acid), which facilitates the passage of the molecule through the lipid layers of the *stratum corneum* and is then "cut off" by special skin enzymes. Transdermal carriers (e.g., liposomes) or other permeability enhancers can also be used for this purpose (Bruno B.J. et al., 2013). In addition, peptides are shorter than proteins and do not form tertiary structures, which are very sensitive to external influences. This makes them easier to preserve in the composition of cosmetic products than larger proteins.

2.1.2. Types of cosmetic peptides

Many cosmetic peptides have been developed and divided into different groups according to the mechanisms and focus of their activities, although they are most actively used in anti-aging procedures. The main groups and their already established and most popular representatives are listed below (Pai V.V. et al., 2017; Schagen S.K., 2017).

Remodeling peptides rejuvenate the composition of the extracellular matrix of the dermis by regulating the natural processes of formation and decay of its components. They can directly affect fibroblasts and thus activate the synthesis of dermal matrix components (matrikins, which are fragments of collagen and elastin and are a signal to fibroblasts that the extracellular matrix is being degraded) or act indirectly through stimulation of growth factors and other ways:
- Matrixyl (INCI: Palmitoyl Pentapeptide-3)
- Ascotide (INCI: Ascorbyl Pentapeptide-3)
- GHK tripeptide as lipoprotein (Dermaxyl et al.), in complex with copper (GHK-Cu), or pure GHK
- SynColl (INCI: Palmitoyl Tripeptide-5)
- Decorinyl (INCI: Tripeptide-10 Citrullin)

Homeostasis-stabilizing peptides activate the skin's own protective potential (including antioxidant protection):
- GHK-Cu (INCI: Prezatide Copper Acetate)
- Kollaren (INCI: Tripeptide-1)
- Peptamide (INCI: Hexapeptide-11)

Melanogenesis-regulating peptides can either enhance or attenuate melanin production mainly by activating or blocking receptors for α-melanocyte stimulating hormone (α-MSH):
- Melatim (INCI: Palmitoyl Tripeptide-30)
- Melitan (INCI: Acetyl Hexapeptide-1)
- Melanostatine (INCI: Nonapeptide-1)

Neurotransmitter peptides (opioid peptides) increase the threshold of skin sensitivity to various external influences (temperature, chemical, mechanical) through the release of opioid mediators and their effect on the cutaneous nerve endings:
- Calmosensine (INCI: Acetyl Dipeptide-1 Cetyl Ester)
- Skinasensil (INCI: Acetyl Tetrapeptide-15)

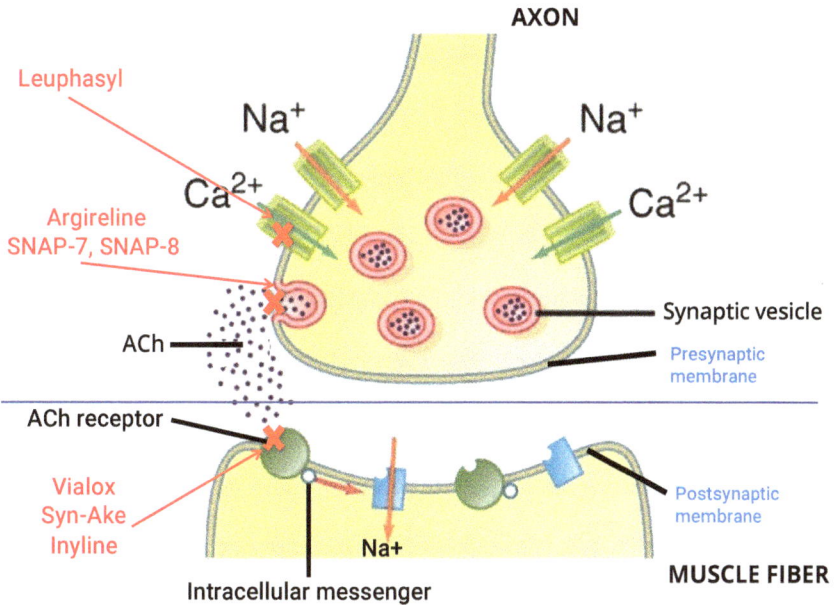

Figure III-2-3. Mechanisms of action of cosmetic myorelaxant peptides at different targets of nerve impulse transmission

The mediator acetylcholine (ACh) enters the synaptic cleft and binds to the acetylcholine receptor (ACh receptor) on the postsynaptic membrane of the muscle cell. This binding results in a release of an intracellular messenger in the muscle, which binds to the inside of the ion channel; the channel opens, and sodium ions enter the cell through it. The signal of muscle fiber contraction is an increase in the sodium ion concentration in the cytoplasm.

Myorelaxant peptides block acetylcholine receptors (in various ways) and thus prevent nerve impulse transmission and muscle fiber contraction (**Fig. III-2-3**). They do not paralyze the muscle like botulinum toxin but rather gently relax it:

- Argirelline (INCI: Acetyl Hexapeptide-3)
- SNAP-7 (INCI: Acetyl Glutamil Hexapeptide-1)
- Syn-Ake (INCI: Dipeptide Diamino Butyroyl Benzylamid Diacetate)
- Vilox (INCI: Pentapeptide-3)

Peptides that improve microcirculation and lymph flow regulate the permeability and improve the elasticity of the vascular wall, have an anti-edema effect, and activate microcirculation:

- Eyeseryl (Acetyl Tetrapeptide-5)

Peptides that act as activators of the antimicrobial peptide production stimulate the formation of their peptide molecules capable of destroying microbial cell membranes:

- Bodyfensine (INCI: Acetyl Dipeptide-3)

Peptides that act as immunomodulators regulate the skin's immune system by normalizing the balance between pro-inflammatory and anti-inflammatory cytokines:

- Rigin (INCI: Palmitoyl Tetrapeptide-3)

This is just a small subset of hundreds of cosmetic peptides. Every year new molecules with new properties are developed.

2.1.3. Growth factors

Growth factors are also conventionally referred to as peptide regulators, although they are larger than peptides. Growth factors belong to a group of cytokines — signaling molecules with the help of which cells send "messages" to each other. They constitute a special group of cytokines and are so named for their ability to stimulate living cell growth, proliferation, and/or differentiation. Due to this feature, growth factors are directly involved in physiological regeneration (natural tissue renewal) and reparation (tissue repair after damage).

The idea of using growth factors for the prevention and treatment of aging signs is based on the fact that, in the skin, even in the absence of visible damage, there are permanent processes of physiological renewal, and this supports its integrity and functional consistency. As a superficial organ, skin is constantly "targeted" by aggressive environmental factors and can be seriously damaged at any time. Therefore, the skin must be in a state of high readiness to repel external attacks and recover quickly after strikes. To do this, all its cellular and extracellular elements should be functional. This is possible due to the precise action coordination with the help of various cytokines and especially growth factors that control the skin tissue renewal processes.

For this reason, preparations containing growth factors are increasingly used in aesthetic medicine. They can be obtained by recombinant methods or extracted from animal tissues (so-called organic preparations). **Regardless of the method and source of production, it is important that the optimal proportion of growth factors in the finished preparation is maintained and there are no by-products** (extractants used at the extraction and purification stage, as well as other inert or, conversely, biologically active molecules without "meaningful" role).

Studies have shown that, in addition to growth factors, it is advisable to include in ready-made preparations substances required for cell metabolism because the nutrient requirements of cells increase during cell growth. Therefore, timely delivery of elementary substances from which the cell synthesizes its own biomolecules is extremely important. Such elementary "building blocks" include:

- **Amino acids** (used for protein synthesis)
- **Oligosaccharides** (polysaccharides are assembled from them, and in addition, they are necessary for energy metabolism)
- **Nucleic acids** (for DNA and RNA synthesis)
- **Fatty acids** (for phospholipids, which are part of cell membranes)

In addition, cells need a set of vitamins and minerals — although these substances are not building material, they are directly involved in metabolic processes in the form of coenzymes, antioxidants, and regulators.

The way of administering such complex physiologically active mixtures is important in terms of clinical effect. Unlike peptides, growth factors are rather large molecules containing dozens of amino acids. The chance of their passage through the intact skin is almost zero, but it increases after the peeling procedure.

Growth factors are increasingly included in cosmetic products. However, recombinant analogs are used for industrial purposes — they are synthesized by bacterial or yeast cells with a fragment of DNA coding for the necessary protein embedded into their genome. **Table III-2-1** shows the recombinant growth factors approved for use in cosmetic products and indicates their names according to the International Nomenclature of Cosmetic Ingredients (INCI).

Table III-2-1. Recombinant (biosynthetic) growth factors in skincare products

INCI NAME	GROWTH FACTOR	APPLICATIONS			
		ANTI-AGING, POST-INJURY RECOVERY	ANTI-PIGMEN-TATION	HAIR CARE	SKIN CALMING
Human oligopeptide-1	Epidermal growth factor	+			
Human oligopeptide-2	Insulin-like growth factor 1	+		+	
Human oligopeptide-3	Basic fibroblast growth factor	+		+	
Human Oligopeptide-4	Thioredoxin	+	+	+	
Human oligopeptide-5	Keratinocyte growth factor	+		+	
Human Oligopeptide-6	Stem cell growth factor			+	
Human oligopeptide-7	Transforming growth factor β3	+	+		
Human oligopeptide-8	Interleukin-10				+
Human oligopeptide-9	Somatotropin (growth hormone)	+			
Human oligopeptide-10	Platelet growth factor	+			
Human oligopeptide-11	Vascular endothe-lial growth factor			+	
Human oligopeptide-12	Fibroblast growth factor 10	+		+	

Continued on p. 115

INCI NAME	GROWTH FACTOR	APPLICATIONS			
		ANTI-AGING, POST-INJURY RECOVERY	ANTI-PIGMEN-TATION	HAIR CARE	SKIN CALMING
Human oligopeptide-13	Acidic fibroblast growth factor	+		+	
Human oligopeptide-14	Transforming growth factor α	+			
Human oligopeptide-15	Interleukin-4				+
Human oligopeptide-16	Timosin-β4	+		+	
Human oligopeptide-18	Noggin			+	
Human oligopeptide-19	Nerve growth factor			+	
Human oligopeptide-20	Tissue inhibitor of metallo-proteinases 2	+			

One of the most frequently asked questions is whether growth factors can stimulate the growth of malignant tumors. However, not a single study on the wound-healing ability of growth factors has yet recorded any cases of malignant cell regrowth.

The main problem with applying growth factors is that they work in the organism as an ensemble, and applying only one growth factor is like trying to obtain symphonic music with, say, a violin or a trombone alone. That is why physiological mixtures of growth factors are the most interesting. They are obtained, in particular, from red blood cells (platelets), amniotic fluid, and placenta extract, as well as tissue and cellular extracts. These include stem cells, or rather, the medium in which they are cultured. However, the question remains about the possibility of their introduction into the skin as a part of cosmetic products — the injection route is more effective here.

2.2. Vitamins

Vitamins (from Latin *vita* — life) are a group of low-molecular-weight organic substances vital to humans and animals in small amounts. Vitamins are not synthesized in the human body and must be taken with food.

All vitamins are used in skincare products, but the frequency of their use varies. **Table III-2-2** shows the most common vitamins in skin and hair care products. Vitamins (more precisely, vitamin-like compounds) include unsaturated fatty acids (vitamin F), bioflavonoids (vitamin P), and lipoic acid (vitamin N). The most widely used are vitamins C, E and B_3 (PP).

Table III-2-2. Vitamins most commonly used in skin and hair care products (most popular are highlighted)

VITA-MIN	CHEMICAL NAME	SOLU-BILITY	FOOD SOURCE	COSMETIC APPLICATIONS
A	Retinol, retinal, carotenoids	f	Retinol: liver, milk Carotenoids: orange-colored fruits, carrots, pumpkin, spinach	• Rejuvenating products • For oily skin and acne-prone skin
B_1	Thiamine	w	Meat (pork), oatmeal, brown rice, vegetables, potatoes, liver, eggs	• For oily skin and acne-prone skin • Lightening products • Anti-inflammatory products • For weak hair
B_2	Riboflavin	w	Dairy products, bananas, corn, green beans, asparagus	• Restorative products • For stressed skin
B_3 (PP)	Niacin, niacinamide	w	Meat, fish, eggs, many vegetables, mushrooms, nuts	• For skin barrier restoration • For stressed, atonic skin • For oily skin • Anti-inflammatory products • Hair regrowth remedies

Continued on p. 117

VITA-MIN	CHEMICAL NAME	SOLU-BILITY	FOOD SOURCE	COSMETIC APPLICATIONS
B_5	Pantothenic acid	w	Meat, broccoli, avocado	• To improve the absorption of other vitamins • Used in a variety of skin and hair care products for general health
B_6	Pyridoxine, pyridoxamine, pyridoxal	w	Meat, vegetables, nuts, bananas	• Anti-hair loss products • Anti-inflammatory products (strengthens skin immunity)
B_7 (H)	Biotin	w	Raw egg yolk, liver, some vegetables, peanuts	• To improve microcirculation • Hair strengthening products
B_9	Folic acid	w	Vegetables (greens), pasta, bread, porridge, liver	• For skin recovery after trauma • Anti-aging products • For improving hair growth and condition
B_{12}	Cyancobala-min, hydroxy-cobalamin, methylcobala-min	w	Meat and other animal products	• For skin recovery after trauma • Hair growth products
C	Ascorbic acid	w	Many fruits and vegetables, liver	Used in a variety of skin-care products
D	Cholecalciferol, ergocalciferol	f	Fish, eggs, liver, mushrooms	Anti-aging products (often together with vitamin A)
E	Tocopherols, tocotrienols	f	Many fruits and vegetables, nuts and seeds	Used in a variety of skincare products
K	Phylloquinone, menaquinones	f	Greens (e.g., spinach), egg yolk, liver	• To improve microcirculation • Anti-cellulite products

Abbreviations: f — fat-soluble, w — water-soluble.

Vitamin C (ascorbic acid)

Vitamin C, an organic compound related to glucose, is one of the main substances in the human diet, and is necessary for the normal functioning of connective and bone tissue. Only one of the isomers, L-ascorbic acid, called vitamin C, is biologically active.

Vitamin C performs the biological functions of a reducing agent and coenzyme of some metabolic processes. It is an antioxidant. In connective tissue (including skin), it takes part in collagen synthesis. It also reduces the activity of melanogenesis and regenerates vitamin E and ubiquinone.

Ascorbic acid is unstable and poorly penetrates the skin, so skincare products usually incorporate ascorbic acid derivatives, such as magnesium ascorbyl phosphate and sodium ascorbyl palmitate. Ascorbic acid is used for photodamaged skin, age-damaged skin with signs of fatigue, and in after-tanning products.

Vitamin E (tocopherol)

Vitamin E contains eight fat-soluble substances, including α- and β-tocopherols and tocotrienols. In skincare, α-tocopherol is used more often. Vitamin E is the body's main fat-soluble antioxidant and is particularly effective in preventing lipid peroxidation. For this reason, vitamin E is considered the main protector of cell membranes and the skin's lipid barrier. Its ability to prevent UV-induced skin damage and reduce inflammation is well documented. When interacting with free radicals, vitamin E is oxidized and loses activity. In the cell, vitamin E is regenerated by vitamin C. Since vitamin C is water-soluble and vitamin E is fat-soluble, these substances must meet at the border of the cell membrane.

Vitamin E is a small lipophilic molecule that easily penetrates and passes through the *stratum corneum*. Some skincare products contain high concentrations of vitamin E. But remember that, by oxidizing, vitamin E becomes a weak radical and can turn from a skin protector into a source of danger, increasing the risk of skin damage.

This raises questions about the usefulness of topical treatments containing high doses of vitamin E. Nevertheless, with judicious and moderate use, vitamin E can significantly strengthen the antioxidant reserves of the skin and prevent skin damage. In the finished product, vitamin E protects lipids from oxidation, preventing spoilage.

Vitamin E is used in care products for mature skin, skin recovery products after tanning, and decorative cosmetics such as lipstick. Natural oils rich in vitamin E, such as wheat germ oil, avocado oil, and walnut oil, are also used.

Vitamin B₃ (niacinamide)

Niacinamide is probably the most versatile cosmetic ingredient. Its main mechanisms of action and effects are presented in **Table III-2-3**.

Table III-2-3. Mechanisms of action of niacinamide and posited associated skin improvements

MECHANISMS OF ACTION	EFFECTS
Inhibition of sebum production (in particular, reduction of diglycerides, triglycerides, and fatty acids)	• Acne reduction • Reducing pore size • Texture enhancement
Stimulation of lipid (ceramides) and protein (keratin, involucrin, filaggrin) synthesis of the epidermal barrier	• Improvement of the skin barrier and hydration • Reducing skin redness • Improvement in rosacea
Anti-inflammatory effect (inhibition of proinflammatory cytokines)	• Anti-aging effect • Reducing skin redness • Improvement in rosacea
Inhibition of melanosome transfer from melanocytes to keratinocytes	Hyperpigmentation reduction
Inhibition of protein glycation via antioxidant effects (niacinamide as a precursor increases the levels of redox cofactors NADH and NADPH), prevention of UV-induced immunosuppression, protective effects of niacinamide against both UVA- and/or UVB-induced DNA damage of melanocytes (in cells, niacinamide-treated cells showed significantly lower numbers of cyclobutane-pyrimidine dimers and 8-oxoG) associated with activation of nucleotide excision repair genes, including sirtuin-1 and p53 genes after UVB exposure, as well as the NRF2 oxidative stress-reducing signaling pathway	Photoprotection

Continued on p. 120

MECHANISMS OF ACTION	EFFECTS
Stimulation of collagen formation and mRNA transcription of some matrix components, associated enzymes, and cytokines: fibulin-1, fibronectin-1, elastin, lysyloxidase (1 and 2), procollagen, collagen (I and III), platelet-derived growth factor beta, actin, connective tissue growth factor, tenascin XB	Wrinkle reduction
Niacinamide can quench the reactive oxygen species produced by PM 2.5 and preventing oxidative damage to DNA, proteins, and lipids. In addition, niacinamide reduces the concentration of intracellular calcium, the amount of which increased under the action of PM 2.5 and serves as a trigger for apoptosis	Anti-pollution

Chapter 3
Depigmenting agents

Methods that directly affect melanogenesis at its various stages are called **depigmenting** or **bleaching methods**. In contrast to depigmenting, lightening methods work differently — they smooth the skin surface by changing its optical properties:

- Exfoliation (chemical peels, microdermabrasion)
- Moistening of the *stratum corneum*
- Filling of wrinkles with cosmetic preparations containing so-called optical pigments, which change the light scattering properties of the skin surface (giving the effect of luminosity and lightening)

Treating pigmentation desorder is a complex task requiring a balanced and patient approach. We have considered all the stages in detail in our *Pigmentation in Cosmetic Dermatology & Skincare Practice* book. We strongly recommend it for anyone who wants to understand this difficult problem and build an optimal treatment scheme. In this book, we focus only on the active ingredients that can be used during the intensive treatment stage in procedures aimed at correcting pigmentation defects. Most of these substances are also suitable for use in home care products, albeit at lower concentrations.

Table III-3-1 shows the main groups of substances found in products used to treat pigmentation, both pharmaceutical and cosmetic. Plant extracts are not listed in the table because they are mixtures of different substances, but they are covered later when we discuss each substance separately.

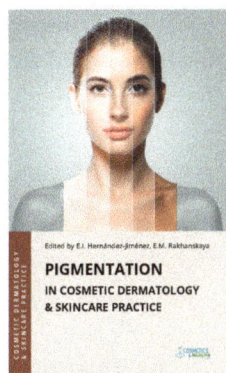

Table III-3-1. The most common ingredients in preparations used to treat pigmentation

MECHANISM OF ACTION	SUBSTANCES
Inhibition of melanogenesis at different stages (true depigmenters)	
Cytotoxic effect	• Hydroquinone • Azelaic acid
Inhibits the synthesis of the amino acid tyrosine from precursors	• N-acetylglycosamine
Tyrosinase inhibition	• Hydroquinone • Arbutin • Kojic acid • Cinnamic acid
Inhibition of melanosome transfer to keratinocytes	• Soybean enzymes • Niacinamide
Reducing agents (prevent oxidative processes, in the course of which melanin is produced)	• Ascorbic acid
Melanosome destruction	• Hydrogen peroxide • Lignin peroxidase
Preventing melanogenesis or reducing its intensity (substances that create conditions conducive for melanocyte activity reduction)	
Binding of metal ions of variable valence (copper, iron), which are initiators of free-radical chain reactions	• EDTA • Azelaic acid • Phytic acid
Reducing inflammation	• Antioxidants (e.g., polyphenols in plant extracts)
Elimination of the consequences of increased melanogenesis (substances that reduce the amount of pigment in the skin by accelerated exfoliation of corneocytes)	
Exfoliating	• Fruit acids (AHAs) • Salicylic acid • Retinol

Currently, trends are moving away from albeit effective but dangerous methods for the health of the skin and the body (e.g., the use of hydroquinone) toward safer modern means and a comprehensive approaches. The most well-known and promising compounds are discussed next.

Azelaic acid

Azelaic acid (1,7-heptandicarboxylic acid) is well-known to dermatologists as a treatment for acne. Studies have shown that it is a weak direct inhibitor of tyrosinase (pronounced inhibition is achieved only in cytotoxic concentrations). However, azelaic acid is characterized by another — indirect — way of action on tyrosinase. It stimulates the activity of the enzyme thioredoxin reductase, which restores oxidized thioredoxin — an endogenous tyrosinase inhibitor. In addition, like hydroquinone, azelaic acid inhibits DNA and RNA synthesis in melanocytes. It is also a chelator of variable valence metal ions (such as iron) that can trigger peroxidation chain reactions and thus activate melanogenesis, and has anti-inflammatory and keratolytic activity.

Arbutin

Arbutin (β-D-glucopyranoside hydroquinone) is a product of hydroquinone glycosylation. It is found in significant amounts in bearberry leaves, which have long been used as a bleaching agent, and in some other plants, although not all of them are characterized by depigmenting action. Blueberries and lingonberries also contain arbutin.

Arbutin attracted the attention of cosmetic manufacturers after experiments showed its ability to inhibit melanin synthesis without having a toxic effect on melanocytes and other skin cells, only slightly reducing melanocyte activity. In human melanoma cell culture, arbutin at a concentration of 0.05 mM significantly reduced tyrosinase activity, and the melanin content in the cells decreased by 39%. However, to achieve the desired effect, therapy with arbutin must last for weeks or even months. But arbutin still has some antioxidant properties and improves skin recovery after photodamage (Zhou H. et al., 2019).

The effectiveness of arbutin as a lightening agent increases with increasing concentration, although too high a concentration can cause increased pigmentation. Synthetic forms of arbutin, α-arbutin and deoxyarbutin, characterized by a more pronounced ability to inhibit tyrosinase, are also used in cosmetic dermatology and skincare (Boo Y.C., 2021). Although there are few independent studies on arbutin, the obtained findings indicate that 3% deoxyarbutin can lighten solar lentigines on light skin, but its effect was negligible on dark skin (Boissy R.E. et al., 2005). There are also encouraging studies on melasma (Zhang Q. et al., 2019).

Kojic acid

Kojic acid (5-hydroxy-2-hydroxymethyl-4-pyrone) is also a tyrosinase inhibitor — it binds to copper in the enzyme and has an exfoliating effect. It can also bind divalent iron ions and intercept free radicals providing antioxidant protection. Among modern bleaching agents, kojic acid rivals hydroquinone and arbutin in popularity but is inferior to them in effectiveness (especially the former). Kojic acid is usually used in 1–4% concentration, as lower concentrations have little or no effect. Often, kojic acid is used in combination with other depigmenting and brightening agents.

The main disadvantage of kojic acid is its potential allergenicity. Therefore, before using kojic acid preparations, a test should be carried out on the elbow bend. At the first sign of irritation, the use should be discontinued.

Ascorbic acid

Ascorbic acid (γ-lactone 2,3-dehydro-L-gulonic acid, vitamin C) is a strong reducing agent, inhibiting melanogenesis by reducing dihydroxyphenylalanine (DOPA) to DOPA-quinone. It also inhibits melanogenesis by interacting with copper ions, which are necessary for melanin synthesis, and blocks the oxidation of 5,6-dihydroxyindole-2-carboxylic acid (DHICA). Nevertheless, for a long time, it was impossible to use ascorbic acid as a bleaching agent since, in its pure form, it is extremely unstable and easily oxidized, while most of its stable analogs do not penetrate the skin well.

Stable forms of ascorbic acid, such as ascorbyl-2-magnesium phosphate and ascorbyl-6-palmitate, are now used in whitening products. Whitening skincare products based on 0.3–3.0% ascorbyl-2-magnesium phosphate are recommended to even out the tone of young skin and improve the condition of aging skin with pigment spots.

An additional advantage of ascorbic acid preparations is their antioxidant activity and ability to stimulate collagen synthesis in the skin. Like all acids, ascorbic acid-based bleaching agents can cause skin irritation.

Niacinamide

Niacinamide (3-pyridine-carboxamide, nicotinamide) is a physiologically active form of vitamin B_3 (niacin, nicotinic acid, vitamin PP). Niacinamide acts by inhibiting the transport of melanosomes into keratinocytes without affecting tyrosinase activity. There is speculation that niacinamide can also affect the cell crosstalk between keratinocytes and melanocytes, whereby keratinocytes begin to signal melanocytes to reduce melanin synthesis. In addition, it has pronounced antioxidant and anti-inflammatory activity, improves skin barrier function by activating the synthesis of keratin, filaggrin, and involucrin, and stimulates fibroblast function (Chhabra G. et al., 2019).

Niacinamide is used in 2–5% concentrations, sometimes in combination with N-acetylglycosamine. The main advantages of niacinamide are its stability and safety. However, its efficacy is lower than that of hydroquinone and kojic acid.

N-acetylglycosamine

Reduces melanin content in melanocytes by inhibiting the conversion of tyrosine precursors to tyrosine. Clinical studies show that 2% N-acetylglycosamine applied for eight weeks reduces facial pigmentation. Usually used in combination with niacinamide, as this combination has a synergistic effect.

Tranexamic acid

Tranexamic acid is a new product in cosmetic dermatology and skincare but has long been known in surgery. It is a synthetic derivative of the amino acid lysine and is used as a styptic, an anti-allergic, and anti-inflammatory agent. Observing patients taking tranexamic acid, experts noticed that their skin became lighter.

Subsequent studies have shown that tranexamic acid influences several targets in the fight against hyperpigmentation — this is already known anti-inflammatory effect — as well as a decrease in the sensitivity of melanocytes to pro-inflammatory agents in general. It also directly inhibits tyrosinase and melanin transfer (Kim M.S. et al., 2015). In addition, tranexamic acid reduces the amount of pro-inflammatory arachidonic acid in keratinocytes, formed in response to UV exposure. It inhibits the production of prostaglandins, thus inhibiting UV-induced melanogenesis and neovascularization (here it mediates inhibition of angiogenic fibroblast growth factor). It can also stimulate melanocyte autophagy (Cho Y.H. et al., 2017). Moreover, tranexamic acid is non-toxic and does not irritate even hypersensitive skin — unlike many de-pigmenting agents (Anju G., 2016).

In a recent study, the efficacy of treating melasma (predominantly mixed) with a 5% tranexamic acid solution and a 3% hydroquinone cream was assessed and compared. The agents were applied once a day for 12 weeks with the mandatory use of sunscreen. The degree of skin lightening was similar in the two groups, but satisfaction was much higher in the tranexamic acid group — due to significantly fewer side effects (Janney M.S. et al., 2019).

Cinnamic acid

Cinnamic acid (β-phenylacrylic acid, benzylidene acetic acid) is a derivative of phenylpropanol which is a precursor of the polyphenol group. It inhibits tyrosinase, has powerful antioxidant properties, and can absorb UVB radiation.

It is used in sunscreens but is a photosensitizer and can cause photoallergic reactions.

Ferulic acid

Ferulic acid is one of the most powerful natural antioxidants. Its strength has been compared to that of superoxide dismutase. Ferulic acid is found in many fruits and plants, such as rice, wheat, oat bran, apples, and coffee beans. Ferulic acid plays a key role in the plants' self-preservation mechanism by strengthening the cell wall and protecting it from microbial damage as well as from sun exposure — it can directly absorb quanta of UVB radiation (Peres D.D. et al., 2018). Therefore, unlike many other compounds, its activity under the sun's influence not only does not diminish but rather increases.

In addition to its pronounced antioxidant, anti-inflammatory, immunomodulatory, and sun protection properties, ferulic acid exhibits some depigmentation activity — it is able to inhibit melanin synthesis and tyrosinase expression. Ferulic acid also stimulates the synthesis of hyaluronic acid, collagen, and tissue inhibitor of metalloproteinase synthesis and inhibits the expression of MMP-1 and MMP-9 (Park H.J. et al., 2018).

Resveratrol

Resveratrol, another powerful antioxidant, was first isolated from dark grapes and grape seeds. In addition to its antioxidant effects, resveratrol can activate the *SIRT1* gene that encodes the sirtuin protein, an enzyme that modifies the histones on which DNA is wound. Through histones, sirtuins can influence the expression of different genes, particularly the *TP53* gene, the activation of which leads to apoptosis. Thus, sirtuins prolong cell life. Resveratrol improves respiratory cell processes and has vasodilatory, anti-allergic, anti-inflammatory, radioprotective, and immunomodulatory effects.

In addition, resveratrol affects several steps in melanogenesis. Being an alternative substrate for tyrosinase, it decreases its melanogenic activity and inhibits transcription of the enzyme. In addition, it reduces UV damage to keratinocytes and inhibits their signaling activity, which, in turn, helps regulate melanocyte function and generally reduces melanin synthesis (Na J.I. et al., 2019).

Fatty acids

Interestingly, unsaturated fatty acids can also regulate melanogenesis. Specifically, oleic, linoleic, and α-linolenic acids inhibit tyrosinase activity and melanogenesis, while palmitic and stearic acids increase it.

Linoleic acid also affects skin pigmentation by stimulating epidermal renewal and increasing the desquamation of cells containing melanin.

Plant extracts with a complex lightening effect

Plant extracts can have a complex lightening effect. For example, some **soybean proteins** inhibit trypsin and serine proteases and exhibit affinity for receptors on the membrane of keratinocytes involved in melanosome transfer. As a result, the transfer of melanosomes from melanocytes to keratinocytes is inhibited, and the skin's pigment content is reduced. Soy extract also has antioxidant and photoprotective activity. The protein fraction of soy extract is used in combination with other lightening agents, retinoids, and sunscreens.

Licorice root extract (licorice, *Glycyrrhyza glabra*) is included in many whitening products. The main components of a licorice root extract that act on pigmentation are glabridine and liquiritin. Glabridine inhibits tyrosinase, and liquiritin acts by increasing the dispersion of melanin. They also have pronounced anti-inflammatory, antimicrobial, and antioxidant properties. Numerous studies have demonstrated their effectiveness against UVB-induced damage and pigmentation (including aggravation of epidermal melasma), which is comparable and, in some cases, superior to hydroquinone (Zubair S., Mujtaba G. et al., 2009; Makino E.T. et al., 2013).

Aloe extract and **mulberry extract** produce a brightening effect by inhibiting tyrosinase and the melanosome tracer. They are also "catchers" of superoxidation radicals and have anti-inflammatory properties. **Shiitake extract** (contains kojic acid) and **green tea extract** (contains polyphenolic compounds with pronounced anti-inflammatory and antioxidant characteristics as well as epigallo-catechin-3-gallate (ECGC) with demonstrated tyrosinase-inhibiting potential) are also used in cosmetic products for pigmented skin.

It should be noted that topical preparations (both drug and skincare products) can be used to lighten ONLY epidermal pigmentation. In the case of dermal pigmentation, energy-based devices can help, but that is a topic for a separate discussion.

Chapter 4
Special care for oily skin

The main tool of intensive care for oily skin is **chemical peeling**, which we discussed above. In particular, for oily skin, salicylic and retinol peels are recommended because they directly affect the sebaceous glands.

For skin with comedones, a manual deep cleansing can be included in the intensive care program. This treatment should be performed after a preliminary steam, a deep saturation of the skin with moisture, and agents that soften sebum and open pores.

Deep cleansing means the **removal (extraction) of comedones**. Whatever we do, whatever drugs or skincare products we use, if the sebaceous gland is clogged, the emergence of inflammation is a matter of time. That is why regular clearing of the sebaceous gland ducts, especially in case of predisposition to acne, is absolutely necessary.

Cleaning begins with forming a passage through which the gland's contents can escape. The classic method of removing closed comedones (**manual extraction**) involves opening the cavity of a clogged pore with a fine needle. Then the skin near the mouth is gently pressed with the fingers. An instrument with one or more holes, an Unna spoon (**Fig. III-4-1**), may be used for extrusion. In the case of large cysts, it may be necessary to curettage the cavity to remove the pus.

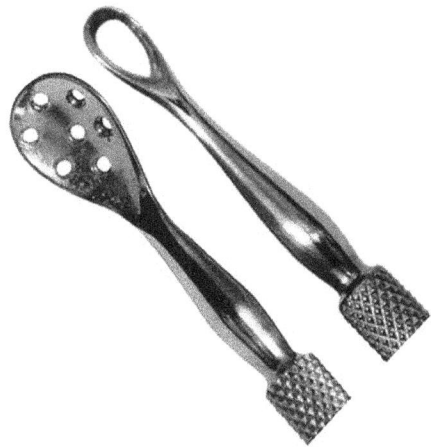

Figure III-4-1. Unna spoon

After cleaning, the skin is treated with antiseptics for several days to avoid infection in the area of the removed comedones.

As for **vacuum extraction**, it cannot guarantee complete comedones removal for obvious reasons, while the risk of damaging the surrounding tissues is high. In addition, it cannot be used in cases of couperosis and increased vascular fragility.

After cleansing, it is possible to use **masks based on clay and mud** — they absorb sebum and have a thermal effect, speeding up the resorption of congestion. But they also absorb water, so after a mud or clay mask, a cream with occlusive components and NMF should always be applied. To avoid over drying the skin, specially prepared cosmetic masks may include lipid components and clay.

Detailed information about skincare products for oily skin and their use is presented in the *Oily Skin, Acne, and Post-Acne in Cosmetic Dermatology & Skincare Practice* book.

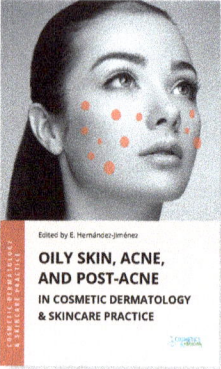

Edited by E. Hernández-Jiménez

OILY SKIN, ACNE, AND POST-ACNE
IN COSMETIC DERMATOLOGY & SKINCARE PRACTICE

Chapter 5
Special care for dry skin

For dry skin, peeling treatment is also indicated — to activate the renewal of the skin barrier. Lactic acid-based peels should be used first because, in addition to their exfoliating effect, as an NMF component, they also ensure skin hydration.

5.1. Lipid replacement therapy

After the first stress caused by damage to the epidermal barrier has passed, **physiological lipids** must be applied — they penetrate deep into the skin, supplying cells with building material. The same preparations are also used in skincare procedures carried out on dry skin but are aimed at solving other aesthetic problems, such as anti-age or toning care, including more conservative methods like exfoliation and massage.

The physiological combination of ceramides (Cer), cholesterol (Ch), and essential free fatty acids (FFA) is considered optimal, i.e., 1:1:1. For atopic dermatitis and some other skin diseases, a formulation of 3 (Cer): 1 (Ch): 1 (FFA) is recommended. For unbalanced nutrition and photodamage, the recommended formulation is 1 (Cer): 1 (Ch) : 3 (FFA). The most rapid restoration of barrier function is observed with these proportions of lipids in the cosmetic composition, regardless of whether a concentrated or diluted lipid mixture is used. Physiological lipids are included in lamellar emulsions, liposomes, and nanocapsules.

Another option is the use of **natural oils**. It would seem to be a good idea, as natural oils do not contain any extraneous chemicals, and many are rich in additional active ingredients such as phytosterols, vitamin E, and carotenoids. However, you should not get addicted to pure oils. Let us remind you that the integrity of the lipid layers of the *stratum corneum* is maintained by the exact ratio of all lipid components — ceramides, cholesterol, and free fatty acids. Oils are inherently neutral fats based on triglycerides. Although they can be broken down into their constituent parts with the release of free fatty acids, they must first penetrate through the lipid layers. Too much oil dilutes the lipid layers, temporarily disrupting their structure. Usually, the structure of the layers is quickly restored. But too frequent application of oils in large amounts can permanently damage the skin barrier function. Everything is good in moderation.

Avocado, rosehip, kukui nut, wheat germ, blackcurrant, evening primrose, and borage oils have proven to be the most physiological in their chemical composition. The last three are especially valuable because they are essential for the skin linolenic acids and contain gamma-linolenic acid, a source of prostaglandin-1, which has a strong anti-inflammatory effect.

In skincare products, natural oils are usually contained in small amounts, so they do not affect the structure of the barrier so noticeably.

5.2. "Deep" moisturizing

The skin can be effectively moisturized with **NMF components**. They penetrate the *stratum corneum* (but not deeper) and increase its water-holding capacity from within — like a sponge that stores moisture. The moisturizing that is felt is usually not as pronounced and does not come as quickly as the "wet compress" effect, but it lasts longer and is less dependent on air humidity.

Hygroscopic "deep" moisturizers include the following substances that can be found in topical products:

- Urea (be careful: it has an irritant potential)
- Amino acids
- Lactic acid and sodium lactate
- Pyroglutamic acid and its sodium salt
- Glycerin
- Sorbitol trioleate
- Glyceret-26
- Methylglucet-20
- Sorbic acid

5.3. Surface moisturizing

High-molecular-weight substances (with a molecular weight of more than 3000 Da) cannot penetrate the *stratum corneum* and remain on its surface, forming a kind of "wet compress" on the skin. This is the principle that works:

- Natural polysaccharides — hyaluronic acid, chondroitin sulfate, pectins
- Proteins of animal and plant origin and their hydrolysates — collagen, elastin, keratin, chitosan
- Polynucleic acids and their hydrolysates
- Propylene glycols (should be avoided for the sensitive skin)

Detailed information about skincare products for dry skin is presented in the *Dry Skin, Atopic Dermatitis, and Psoriasis in Cosmetic Dermatology & Skincare Practice* book.

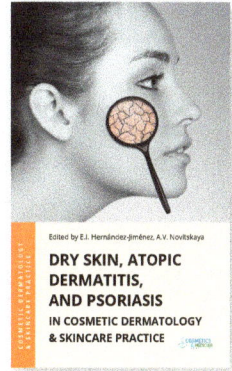

Edited by E.I. Hernández-Jiménez, A.V. Novitskaya

DRY SKIN, ATOPIC DERMATITIS, AND PSORIASIS
IN COSMETIC DERMATOLOGY & SKINCARE PRACTICE

Part IV

Post-treatment skincare

Often, the final stage determines whether the procedure will end smoothly or complications will arise. At this stage, it is better not to load the skin with active substances and use only what is necessary.

Almost any intensive cosmetic procedure involves "opening up" the skin, partial or complete destruction of its barrier structures and, in many cases, induces direct skin damage. No active ingredients can be delivered to the skin without breaching the skin barrier, but once the goal has been reached, every effort must be made to get the skin's barrier and protective systems back in a peaceful mode of functioning. This is accomplished with moisturizers, as well as soothing, anti-inflammatory, antioxidant, microbiome-restoring, and sunscreen products. It should be noted that most of these components also form the basis of home care.

Before turning to specific recommendations, let's list what these groups of ingredients include.

Chapter 1
Cosmetic ingredients

1.1. Moisturizers

To ensure that your skin is fully hydrated, let's remember the basic water-holding structures of the *stratum corneum*.

1. **Sebum (natural emollient)** — smooths horny scales, reducing the area of contact between intercellular spaces and the air (consequently reducing the area from which evaporation occurs). It creates an additional waterproof layer on the skin, which prevents transepidermal water loss (TEWL). When the triglycerides of sebum are broken down by *Cutibacterium*, which infest the sebaceous gland ducts, glycerin is released, which binds water from the atmosphere and holds it in the *stratum corneum* and on its surface.

2. **Lipid structures (lipid barrier)** fill in the intercellular spaces of the *stratum corneum* and control diffusion of water molecules and water-soluble substances (in other words, they regulate TEWL).

3. **NMF** is a complex of low-molecular-weight hygroscopic molecules (free amino acids, urea, lactic acid, sodium pyroglutamate). They are concentrated mainly near the corneocytes and create a water shell around them.

4. **Keratin** is a large protein that fills corneocytes. It is insoluble but, like all proteins, swells in water and firmly binds water molecules by electrostatic bonds.

When one or more water-holding structures are disturbed (deficient, structurally altered), the water level in the *stratum corneum* declines. As we mentioned above, restoration of barrier function is important for all skin types and all aesthetic conditions. Different approaches can be adopted to increase skin hydration. In addition to physiological lipids and moisture catchers, occlusive and sebum-mimicking topical formulations are used.

The **occlusive** and **sebum-mimicking preparations** create a semi-permeable surface film that prevent TEWL. This increases water concentration in the *stratum corneum*. The natural occlusive film is sebum. Oxygen and carbon dioxide pass through it freely, and water evaporation is inhibited thanks to the smoothing of corneocytes and the glycerin present in sebum. The latter also has a mild "enveloping" effect that reduces the sensitivity of nerve endings, which is also important for hypersensitive skin. Cosmetic ingredients that mimic sebum and slow down water evaporation include:

- Mineral oil, petrolatum (vaselinum), liquid paraffin, and ceresin — hydrocarbons, petroleum substances
- Liquid silicones (silicone oils) — hydrophobic high-molecular-weight organosilicon compounds
- Lanolin — wax substance obtained from animal wool
- Natural waxes and their esters, such as beeswax, vegetable waxes (e.g., pine wax, cane wax)
- Animal fats (goose fat, spermaceti, pork fat, badger fat, etc.)
- Squalene and its derivative squalane — natural compounds of human sebum, obtained from shark liver and some plants
- Vegetable oils (mostly refractory — so-called cosmetic butters, such as shea butter and cocoa butter)

It is important to note that some emollients are comedogenic, i.e., they are able to provoke the formation of comedones, especially in oily skin. Comedogenic compounds include isopropyl palmitate, isopropyl myristate, butyl stearate, isopropyl isostearate, decyl oleate, isostearyl neopentanoate, isostearyl stearate, myristyl myristate, and cocoa butter. But petroleum jelly and paraffin, contrary to the popular opinion, do not provoke comedones.

1.2. Antioxidants

Antioxidants are natural or synthetic oxidation inhibitors that can slow down oxidation. An antioxidant can lower ROS levels and prevent

In a reduction–oxidation (redox) reaction, an electron transfer occurs from the reducing agent (electron donor) to the oxidizing agent (electron acceptor)

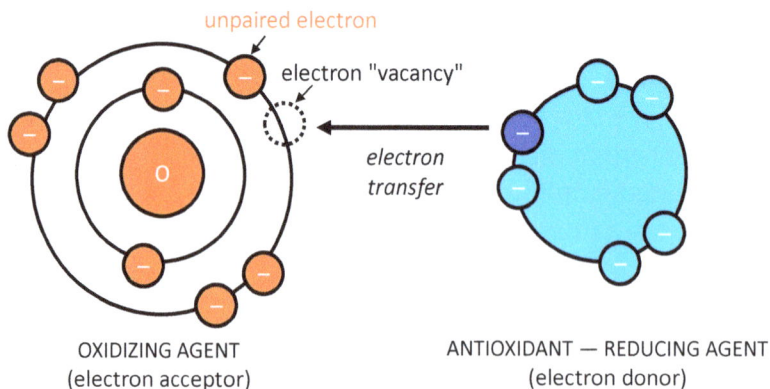

Figure IV-1-1. The antioxidant gives its electron to the free radical, thereby reducing it to a stable form

free radical chain reactions. Usually, an antioxidant sacrifices itself, i.e., it reacts with ROS, turning it into a chemically stable and inactive molecule. In doing so, the antioxidant becomes a free radical but is much less reactive (**Fig. IV-1-1**). In this form, it is not dangerous to the environment but is also non-functional unless it is restored to its active state. Thus, **the antioxidant molecule, once reacted, loses its antioxidant power**.

Our body synthesizes most antioxidants on its own, replenishing them as needed, but some of them (e.g., vitamin C, flavonoids, selenium) come from food. However, they are often quite actively depleted by external factors.

Antioxidants differ in their potency, targets, and mechanisms of action. In addition, some are fat-soluble and "work" in the lipid phase (in membranes, preventing lipid peroxidation), while others are water-soluble and protect water-phase compounds from free-radical attacks. **The greatest antioxidant effect is achieved when antioxidants act in pairs or even groups.** After giving its electron to a free radical, the antioxidant is oxidized and becomes inactive. To get it back to its working state, it has to be restored again. For example, glutathione restores vitamin C, and vitamin C restores vitamin E.

Popular cosmetic antioxidants:

- Vitamin C
- Vitamin E
- β-Carotene
- α-Lipoic acid (thioctic acid)
- Coenzyme Q_{10} (ubiquinone)
- *Maritime pine* bark extract (known as Pycnogenol®)
- Resveratrol
- Lactobionic acid
- Green tea extract
- Açai berry extract
- *Polypodium leucotomos* fern extract
- *Centella asiatica* extract
- *Boswellia serrata* extract

1.3. Soothing and calming agents

Ingredients with anti-inflammatory and soothing properties can help reduce inflammation and calm the skin. Some plant extracts rich in polyphenols and antioxidants (chamomile, aloe, *Centella asiatica*, and many others), which are traditionally popular cosmetic ingredients, have these properties. A little more information about some of them is given below.

The new and promising developments in skin hypersensitivity treatment include inhibition of the activity of the transient receptor potential cation channel subfamily V (TRPV) responsible for the perception of various types of irritants by synthetic peptides (Skinasensyl™ and Calmosensine™) and *Albatrellus ovinus* extract.

1.4. Substances that normalize the skin microbiome

A modern and very promising strategy is the use of skincare products that are friendly to the skin microbiome. The following types of ingredients are used for this purpose:

1. **Probiotics** — live microorganisms that, when used in sufficient quantities, positively affect human health

2. **Prebiotics** — selectively fermented media that positively affect the skin (a "feed" for bacteria)
3. **Synbiotics** — combination of microorganism with its nutrient medium

Live **probiotics** are almost impossible to introduce into the cosmetic formula since it is necessary to provide conditions for preserving the vital activity of "good" microorganisms while preventing the reproduction of "undesirable" microorganisms. Therefore, bacterial biomass is processed — e.g., lysed, fermented — to destroy them and collect useful compounds. Bacterial fragments interact with the receptors of skin cells, enhancing local immunity and production of anti-inflammatory factors, and can also play the role of nutrients for other bacteria (i.e., act as probiotics).

As for **prebiotics** per se, scientists have gone to great lengths to create a "nutrient base" that stimulates saprophytic bacteria but not pathogenic and opportunistic microflora. Typical prebiotics include inulin, fructooligosaccharides, galactooligosaccharides, and lactulose. Gradually, xylooligosaccharides, long-chain β-glucans, and glucomannan were added.

Examples of synbiotics include the most commonly used combinations:

- inulin + *Lactobacillus*
- xylooligosaccharides + *Lactobacillus*, *Streptococcus* and *Bifidobacterium*
- lactosucrose + *Lactobacillus* and *Bifidobacterium*

The efficacy of pre- and probiotics in treating skin disorders is currently being actively studied, and the results are impressive. For example, topical application of a cream containing *Lactobacillus plantarum* to acne-prone skin reduces the number of inflammatory elements and erythema, and topical application of lysates of *Vitreoscilla filiformis* reduces inflammation and significantly improves the course of atopic and seborrheic dermatitis compared to placebo (Muizzuddin N. et al., 2012; Mottin V.H.M., Suyenaga E.S., 2018). A cream containing extract of *Bifidobacterium longum* decreased the reactivity of hypersensitive skin under experimental conditions (Guéniche A. et al., 2010).

There are reports that glucooligosaccharides are successfully used in controlling the number of *Staphylococcus aureus* in skin affected by atopic dermatitis (Blanchet-Réthoré S. et al., 2017). Various formulations with β-glucans have improved wound healing processes, decreased skin dryness, and reduced itching in bacterial infections (Kiousi D. E. et al., 2019).

An important factor in probiotic skincare products is the ability to maintain the pH level on the skin surface.

1.5. UV filters and anti-pollution agents

UV filters are the main substances in any sunscreen formula. They are divided into two groups according to their mechanism of action (**Table IV-1-1**):
1) **physical** — reflect and scatter UV rays
2) **chemical** — absorb UV rays and transform the absorbed energy into heat

1.5.1. Chemical UV filters

The most "powerful" **chemical UV filters** are synthesized organic substances (e.g., benzophenones, cinnamates, salicylates, camphor, and para-aminobenzoic acid derivatives). Substances of natural origin provide less effective UV protection — these are plant pigments that can absorb UV radiation (e.g., caffeic acid). Natural UV filters are introduced in formulations as auxiliary ingredients to attract customers that prefer natural cosmetics.

However, there are nuances to chemical filters, as many have irritating potential even for people with healthy skin, as they decompose when exposed to the sun and can form potentially toxic compounds.

Particular caution is needed if using older filters such as benzophenone-3 (aka Oxybenzone), benzophenone-4, para-aminobenzoic acid (PABA), avobenzone, and octocrylene, which have irritating and other potentially negative effects (Diffey B., 2020). The new Tinosorb S filters have undergone much more research before entering the market and are considered much more stable and safer. Moreover, they protect against a wide range of radiation.

Table IV-1-1. UV filters: action, properties, and representatives

	CHEMICAL FILTERS	PHYSICAL FILTERS
Chemical nature	Organic compounds	Inorganic particles (< 1 µm)
Mechanism of action	Absorb UV rays with subsequent release of heat (infrared radiation)	Reflect and scatter UV rays
Distribution in the skin	On the surface and within the *stratum corneum*	On the surface of the *stratum corneum*
Penetration	Very low	No penetration
Benefits	• High level of photoprotection • Possibility to create combinations with minimal "working" concentrations and a wide protective spectrum • Good "cosmetic" • Good compatibility with other formulation components	• High level of photoprotection • UVA/B protection • Inertness against UV rays
Disadvantages	Potential phototoxicity due to phototransformation upon UV absorption (approved substances have successfully passed long-term safety tests, so the risks here are close to zero)	• "The whitewash effect" • Precipitation • Difficulties when combined with some other components of the formulation • Quite high "working" concentrations
UV filters approved for use in cosmetics in the EC:		
INCI and trade names (in parentheses)		
UVA filters (400–315 nm)	• Avobenzone (Parsol 1789) • Bisdisulizole disodium (Neo Heliopan AP) • Diethylamino hydroxybenzoyl hexyl benzoate (Uvinul A Plus) • Ecamsule (Mexoryl SX)* • Methyl anthranilate	—

Continued on p. 143

	CHEMICAL FILTERS	PHYSICAL FILTERS
UVB filters (315–290 nm)	• 4-Aminobenzoic acid (PABA) • Cinoxate • Ethylhexyl triazone (Uvinul T 150) • Homosalate • 4-Methylbenzylidene camphor (Parsol 5000) • Octyl methoxycinnamate (Octinoxate) • Octyl salicylate (Octisalate) • Padimate O (Escalol 507) • Phenylbenzimidazole sulfonic acid (Ensulizole) • Polysilicone-15 (Parsol SLX) • Trolamine salicylate	—
UVA/V filters	• Bemotrizinol (Tinosorb S) • Benzophenones 1–12 • Dioxybenzone • Drometrizole trisiloxane (Mexoryl XL)* • Iscotrizinol (Uvasorb HEB) • Octocrylene • Oxybenzone (Benzophenone-3) • Sulisobenzone	• Titanium dioxide • Zinc oxide • Cerium oxide/dioxide **Hybrid (chemical/physical):** • Bisoctrizole (Tinosorb M)

* The Mexoryl UV filters® SX and XL are patented by L'Oréal and are found only in their products.

1.5.2. Physical UV filters

Physical UV filters include micronized insoluble particles of titanium dioxide (Ti_2O) and zinc oxide (ZnO). They have an excellent safety profile and protect the skin from a wide range of UV radiation. However, there is one limitation: the microparticles stain the skin white. This "whitening effect" can be combated by reducing the size of the particles, e.g., to nano-size. But there is another serious problem: when exposed to UV radiation, very small titanium dioxide particles become photocatalysts and can initiate chemical reactions between the other ingredients in the preparation. To prevent this undesirable effect, the surface of the particles is modified by applying a special polymer coating.

UV filters based on cerium (Ce) — phosphates and oxides/dioxides — have also been developed. Comparing the photoprotective properties of cerium oxide with titanium dioxide and zinc dioxide shows even more pronounced filter efficiency. However, despite the initial hopes of non-toxicity, cerium oxide nanoforms are also characterized by potent cytotoxicity and pro-oxidant activity (Miri A. et al., 2020), as are nanoforms of other physical filters. However, micronized forms of all these filters are currently considered the safest.

For the product to provide the declared photoprotection — SPF for UVB protection, Persistent Pigment Darkening (PPD) or Protection Grade of UVA (PA) index for UVA protection — we recommend applying 2 mg/cm^2 at two-hour intervals (or more frequently if skin was exposed to water). Unfortunately, the average consumer uses a smaller amount of the product — about 0.5 mg/cm^2. As a result, the promised sun protection is at least four times weaker. Still, it's important to remember that SPF is not a guarantee but only a guideline for choosing a product, so the best sunscreen is clothing, hat, and shade.

Sunscreen formulations include substances that give the finished product additional properties, such as moisturizing components, anti-inflammatory agents, antioxidants (usually fat-soluble vitamin E), and even immunomodulators (yeast polysaccharides, chitosan). But the main thing here is not to overdo it. There is a general rule: **the higher the degree of photoprotection, the fewer additional "active" substances the formulation should contain**. There is a reason for that: sunscreen with a high photoprotection factor should restrain the "pressure" of ultraviolet light for a long time, which means that anything that can potentially increase the photosensitivity of the skin should be avoided. Of course, fragrances and colorants are also highly undesirable, especially in the case of sensitive skin.

Another nuance is the introduction of anti-inflammatory agents into sunscreens. Since the only sign of severe photodamage is the appearance of erythema, and they "take it away," there are concerns that their inclusion in the formulation may give people a false sense of security — "Since my skin is not red yet, the sunscreen is working, and I am protected" — when that may not be the case at all.

On the other hand, the use of photostable antioxidants in the formula is welcome. Not only do they not reduce the sun protection capacity of the product, but they also increase skin protection from free radicals formed under the influence of UV radiation. Vitamin E directly protects DNA from undergoing typical UV-induced mutations under the influence of free radicals (Delinasios G.J. et al., 2018).

1.5.3. Protection from visible light

As for **protection from visible light**, the high-intensity blue light that can lead to pigmentation in people with skin phototypes III and darker is only provided by reflecting or scattering light. Inorganic sunscreens, primarily iron oxide but also titanium dioxide or zinc oxide, can help because their reflectance is in the UV to the visible spectrum. In addition, blue light, like **infrared light**, can provoke the generation of free radicals, which can be prevented with the use of antioxidants (Sondenheimer K., Krutmann J., 2018).

Ideally, it is better to avoid sun exposure between 10:00 a.m. and 04:00 p.m. when there is peak solar activity. It should also be noticed that in the mountains, in the presence of reflective surfaces (snow, water), exposure to UV rays increases. Once again, the best sunscreens are clothes, a hat, and shade.

1.5.4. Anti-pollution protection

Another line of defense is **against environmental pollutants**: particulate matter (PM), organic compounds, oxides of nitrogen, sulfur, and carbon. Environmental pollution is a big problem in cities and especially in megacities, and some scientists believe it also contributes to the rapid increase in the sensitive skin incidence.

Studies have shown that most pollutants trigger oxidative stress and inflammation in the skin (Parrado C. et al., 2019). Therefore, antioxidant and anti-inflammatory agents are currently the main anti-pollution substances (see Part IV, sections 1.2 and 1.3).

Chapter 2
Cosmetic products to complete the procedure

It would be great if we could explain to our skin that we are doing cosmetic procedures for its good. However, the skin's main function is protective, so very often, the skin perceives all external manipulations as aggression.

This is true even when applying nourishing skin cream. From the skin cells' perspective, anything trying to penetrate skin's surface (except oxygen) is a potential enemy. Creams can contain emulsifiers that break down the protective barrier, plant extracts, animal proteins that can turn out to be allergens, and oils that potentially upset the delicate balance of skin lipids. What about when we have to damage the skin in order to remove its worn structures, as is the case with peels, invade its biochemical processes by inhibiting enzyme activity or changing the synthetic activity of cells (bleaching, fat splitting), pierce the skin's protective layer with needles (microneedling, mesotherapy, dermal fillers) or inject toxins into it (botulinum toxin)?

If you take the skin cells' point of view, you'll see that they have every reason to sound the alarm. That's exactly what they do after a cosmetic procedure. It means that any aggressive and potentially dangerous factor can provoke a "military conflict," primarily by releasing inflammatory mediators — free radicals appearing in the skin due to immune system cell activity and increased melanocyte activity. At the same time, it is important to realize that many treatments aimed to enhance skin regeneration and renewal work on the principle of controlled damage — both inflammation and free radicals (to some extent) are necessary to achieve this goal. Therefore, the challenge is to allow these processes to develop, keeping them under control and not creating an explosive situation.

The final stage of the cosmetic procedure is designed with the following in mind:

- Skin type and condition
- Peculiarities of the procedure performed
- Degree of damage to the skin's protective barrier
- Goals of intensive exposure

2.1. Post-peeling care

Chemical peeling refers to methods of controlled skin damage and is inevitably accompanied by partial or complete destruction of the protective barrier. As is easy to understand, the increased alertness of skin cells combined with a weakened or destroyed barrier creates an explosive situation.

The following undesirable phenomena may occur immediately after the procedure:

- Itching
- Burning
- Redness
- Edema
- Eye irritation and lacrimation (if the procedure is performed around the eyes)

After a few days, weeks, or even in the longer term, complications may occur and usually manifest as:

- Infection on the background of a compromised barrier — especially in people with a weak immune system and endocrine abnormalities
- Acneiform lesions — teenagers, mentally unstable people
- Scarring, delayed healing, skin texture disorders — people with endocrine disorders adhering to different diets after an illness
- Dyschromia (hyper-, hypopigmentation) — people with genetically dark skin and increased basic melanocyte activity are at risk

Even after superficial peeling, the skin's defenses are weakened, so the primary tasks immediately after the procedure and in the early post-peel stage of recovery are:

1) **minimize the effect of aggressive external factors and water evaporation by creating an artificial barrier on the skin** — UV protection, occlusion
2) **keep the inflammatory process under control** — by using anti-inflammatory and soothing agents

During rehabilitation, physiological lipids and emollient-based preparations and non-contact physical therapy, such as low-level laser (light) therapy (LLLT), are best.

2.1.1. Calming agents

Although in clinical practice drugs are used to fight inflammation, many have serious side effects and cannot be used for long. In cosmetic dermatology and skincare, instead of drugs, natural substances that modulate inflammation — modify the processes in such a way that the damage is minimal — are thus preferred.

For example, free radicals play a major role in inflammation. Some immune system cells produce hydrogen peroxide and other ROS against infection, which can provoke a cascade of free-radical oxidation reactions in the skin. Therefore, to prevent excessive tissue damage during inflammation, the skin's antioxidant system can be supported with cosmetic antioxidants (see Part IV, section 1.3).

Other substances change the set of signaling molecules that cells produce during inflammation. They do this by slightly modifying the direction of chemical processes. This group includes oils rich in essential fatty acids (precursors of immune system regulatory molecules — prostaglandins) as well as substances of plant origin that inhibit the activity of metalloproteinases (enzymes responsible for collagen destruction) and the production of pro-inflammatory cytokines and nitric oxide. The difference between such natural substances and medications is that they act gently and, in most cases, do not affect normal physiological processes in healthy skin.

Since after peeling, the skin's protective barrier is broken, only preparations free of irritants and destroyers can be applied to the skin. It can be a soothing gel mask with polysaccharides and extracts of plants known in folk medicine or used in food (e.g., chamomile, aloe, calendula). While oriental medicine consists of an entire arsenal of useful remedies, the *Centella asiatica* (Gotu kola) should be highlighted. In Ayurvedic and Chinese medicine, centella is often used to treat various skin disorders (infections, wounds, ulcers, and even leprosy), and respiratory diseases, for blood pressure reduction and nervous system boosting. Modern science approves its use in wound care. Experiments have shown that wound epithelialization is accelerated after treatment with centella extract. In addition, centella extract exhibits immunomodulatory activity and reduces inflammation. As centella contains a group of active substances called asiaticosides, studies have confirmed that they can induce skin fibroblasts to produce more collagen, improving skin elasticity.

Purified plant polysaccharides such as aloe vera, P-glucans, and fucoidans of brown seaweed exhibit anti-inflammatory and immunomodulatory activity. Brown seaweed fucoidans not only regulate the inflammatory response (as confirmed in allergic skin models) but also stimulate skin renewal processes by increasing the production of collagen, elastin, and glycosaminoglycans, making them the ideal anti-inflammatory ingredient in post-peeling care.

Formulations containing an effective concentration of one, two, or three plants work better and are less likely to cause skin irritation than those containing many different extracts. Essential oils should be avoided, as many are potential allergens and skin irritants.

Cooling the skin with cold compresses or ice also helps to soothe it.

2.1.2. Occlusive agents

Care must be taken to prevent excessive water loss in all cases where the skin's protective barrier is damaged. The greater the damage, the faster the skin must be "locked up." Otherwise too much water evaporation provokes the release of inflammatory mediators, leading to itching, redness, and swelling and potentially hyperpigmentation. Therefore, products with an occlusive effect are necessary after medium-depth or deep chemical peeling. The occlusive agents quickly "calm" the skin and prevent the development of an inflammatory reaction in response to the sudden destruction of the barrier structures. Subsequently, you can start applying products to help restore the barrier, but in those first minutes and hours after the peeling, the task is very simple: to close the skin and block the alarms. Petrolatum-based occlusive ointments are often the easiest solution to this problem, as they are biologically inert, do a good job, and have a long history of use. The ointments may contain analgesic additives.

After superficial peeling that not accompanied by significant damage to the barrier, a moisturizing cream with aloe gel, hyaluronic acid, and other natural polymers would usually suffice. In this case, achieving complete occlusion is unnecessary as the aim is to ensure that the skin does not lose moisture and is not exposed to potential irritants. Products based on lamellar and liposomal emulsions, which effectively close the gaps in the barrier, are useful at this stage.

2.1.3. Sun protection

The sun, so pleasantly caressing the skin, gives life to all the inhabitants of our planet, helps our skin to synthesize vitamin D, enhances the regeneration processes, and simply cheers up our mood. But after chemical peeling, we must forget about sunbathing for a while. The skin, "opened" by the peeling procedure and in a state of full alertness, will react to UV radiation with a dramatic increase in melanocyte activity, which may lead to unwanted pigmentation. Ingredients such as AHA directly increase the skin's sensitivity to UV radiation — this should always be remembered.

When choosing a sunscreen, both the skin phototype and the peculiarities of the treatment should be considered.

For example, if we were talking about a trip to the sea, we would say that dark skin has a sufficiently high level of melanin, and using products with high SPF for this skin is unjustified. However, for sun protection after chemical peeling, the opposite is true. Scientific evidence indicates that melanocytes react not only to UV radiation but also to ROS and inflammatory mediators in the skin. Any damage to keratinocytes can lead to melanocyte activation. Since dark skin has been formed under constant exposure to intense UV radiation, heat, and drastic fluctuations in humidity (from dry to rainy seasons), melanocytes produce large quantities of pigment but are also very stubborn, vigorous, and highly combative. Consequently, the risk of developing hyperpigmentation in such skin is very high. After chemical peeling, and even more so after laser resurfacing and dermabrasion, the patient is advised to avoid the sun.

For people with fair and sensitive skin, it is very important that the sunscreen does not irritate the skin, so it is advisable to use a product with physical or modern chemical filters. At the same time, it should provide sufficient protection, although most people do not apply sunscreen in sufficient amount or as frequently as they should. That is why we recommend using products with a high protection factor (SPF 50, RA+++). For people with sensitive skin, it is recommended to use sunscreens with an UV index of 2 and higher. This index describes the sun's intensity and is broadcast by many resources and apps for a particular zone and season — accordingly, it is always possible to pick up individual sun protection. Since no sunscreen can provide 100% protection from skin damage, the client should be advised to avoid the sun during recovery. Sunscreens protect the skin in the same way that a safety net protects an acrobat in a circus: they minimize the risk but do not eliminate it completely.

Sunscreen for post-peel care should be easy to spread, not sticky, not leave a greasy shine, and not irritate the skin. This can be achieved with the use of a moisturizing day cream with an SPF of about 15 in combination with a mineral powder with UV filters. Modern mineral powders have a thin, lightweight texture and usually contain Ti_2O and/or ZnO. This double protection makes it possible to considerably reduce the amount of UV filters in the cream and thus reduces the risk of skin irritation.

2.2. After treating pigmented skin

Intense skin whitening procedures (excluding peeling) do not damage the barrier much, so occlusion is not necessary immediately afterward. At the end of the procedure, antioxidants and herbal extracts are applied to the skin to prevent inflammation. Before going out in the daytime, sunscreen should be applied. These same products are also used for in-home care.

It should be remembered that some plant extracts can exhibit photodynamic effects (e.g., St. John's wort), i.e., increase pigmentation if the skin is exposed to UV rays. Sunscreens should contain broad-spectrum UV filters, and the SPF should be high enough to almost block the sun's rays completely.

Plant extracts exhibiting antioxidant, anti-inflammatory, and brightening properties include licorice, mulberry, green tea, shiitake mushroom, bearberry, raspberry, aloe, ginseng, and wild yam (see Part IV, sections 1.2 and 1.3). Raspberries contain tiliroside, an organic substance that inhibits tyrosinase activity and melanocyte synthetic activity. In addition, raspberries have anti-inflammatory and antioxidant properties. Aloe contains the brightening ingredient aloesin along with the immunomodulatory polysaccharide acemannan suppressing inflammation. Wild yam contains diosgenin, which reduces melanogenesis, as well as phytoestrogens, which have anti-inflammatory effects and improve mature skin.

UV filters, antioxidants, and plant extracts with anti-inflammatory and melanogenesis-suppressing effects significantly increase the effectiveness of skin-lightening treatments.

2.3. After treating oily or dry skin

In the case of non-aggressive treatments that do not require recovery and protection, completing the session with cream for your skin type and sunscreen during intense sun exposure is recommended. The most important part of a successful beauty treatment, or rather a course of treatments, is home care, which is discussed in the next part.

Part V

In-home skincare

1.1. Aims of in-home care

Imagine that you went to the gym and spent two hours working hard on the machines. Your muscles feel good, you feel great, and you are proud of the time you spent productively. Now imagine that your next visit to the club will happen in a few months or even years, and in between, you will be lying on the couch in front of the TV. No matter how intensive your workout is, it is useless if you don't keep yourself in shape.

Skincare is similar. For cosmetic procedures to bring maximum benefit with minimal risk of unwanted side effects, they need to be complemented (or, as experts say, supported) by competent in-home care. In-home care is especially important during the recovery period after chemical peels and other aggressive procedures, as it can speed up skin recovery, reduce the risks, and greatly improve the procedure's effectiveness.

The aims of in-home care after cosmetic procedures are:
1. Prevention of possible adverse events
2. Support for skin repair
3. Improvement of the cosmetic treatment effects
4. Creation of optimal conditions for the functioning of skin cells
5. Preparation of the skin for subsequent procedures

These aims are closely related to each other. Thus, by creating comfortable conditions for cell life, the risks of unwanted side effects are reduced, while the desired effects are enhanced.

Increasing the skin's reparative potential is crucial for the success of future cosmetic procedures, especially if they involve skin damage.

1.2. After the in-salon treatment

Post-treatment care depends on not only the condition of the skin but also the specifics of the intensive impact on the skin. It is no coincidence that the manufacturers of professional skincare products to be used in-salon treatment develop products for supporting home care.

1.2.1. After the chemical peeling

Ideally, in-home care should begin even before the peeling treatment. At this stage, preparations with cosmetic retinoids (retinol and its esters) or AHAs in low concentrations are used to even out and thin the *stratum corneum* and activate the cell renewal processes of the epidermis to increase its regenerative potential. The use of cosmetic retinoids must be discontinued at least two weeks before the peeling. In the pre-peel period, products that inhibit melanocyte activity and antioxidant compounds are also recommended to enhance the skin's antioxidant mechanisms to counteract the inevitable oxidative stress after the peeling. It would also be useful to "feed" the skin with physiological lipids. All this can be compared to the preparation for sports competitions. For your skin to "perform" successfully, it needs to get in perfect shape.

After peeling, the skin enters a period of healing, which is not much different from the wound healing process. The damaged skin exfoliates intensively, which is often accompanied by itching. If the peeling is aggressive enough, an inflammatory process can unfold in the skin, usually accompanied by increased generation of free radicals, activation of proteolytic enzymes, and changes in vascular permeability and tone (edema, redness). From the first days, the skin starts intensive regeneration — there is an increased cell division of the basal layer, new proteins are actively synthesized, and capillaries are growing. During this period, skin cells are like residents of a city that has experienced a natural disaster. If they are enthusiastic, mobilize their resources, and work together to clear debris, restore communications, and rebuild destroyed homes, sooner or later, the city will be rebuilt and will look better than before. However, if they suffer from hunger and thirst, fall into despondency, or start blaming each other, reconstruction will be very slow, and full recovery will not happen. Therefore, during this period, it is very important to prevent infection, ensure adequate hydration and uninterrupted supply of skin-building materials, and create a favorable psychological background.

Once the initial reactions (if any) have subsided and the barrier function is at least partially restored, you can begin a program of remodeling — so called structural changes in the skin, during which its rejuvenation takes place. To do this, the following must be kept in mind.

1. **Improvement of microcirculation.** A good blood supply is a basic prerequisite for successful skin repair. Skin cells may not receive the necessary oxygen and nutrients without an adequate blood supply. The importance of a good blood supply is demonstrated by the example of pressure sores, where stagnant blood circulation leads to long-term non-healing ulcers. The blood supply to the skin deteriorates with age, so older individuals need to pay more attention to this issue. In addition, good vascular tone reduces the risk of persistent redness and excessive edema. Exercise and extracts of ginkgo, horse chestnut, needle comfrey, and some peptides, such as copper-containing peptides, improve microcirculation.

2. **Restore the water balance.** Sufficient moisture in the skin is necessary for the rapid migration of signaling molecules. In addition, severe dehydration creates additional stress and can intensify the inflammatory processes.

3. **Delivery of essential omega-3 and omega-6 acids to the skin.** Omega-6 acids are needed to rebuild the protective barrier, while omega-3 acids are used to synthesize prostaglandins that keep inflammation in check.

4. **Antioxidant protection.** Inflammation is accompanied by generation of ROS, which creates conditions for oxidative stress and skin damage. However, we should also remember that some ROS are necessary to stimulate skin regeneration, so do not "overdo" antioxidants either. A better solution is to use plant extracts with complex action. For example, green tea extract contains polyphenolic antioxidants, and has anti-inflammatory and brightening properties.

5. **Suppression of melanogenesis.** As any peeling is a stress for the skin, it responds by mobilizing all defense systems, includ-

ing melanocyte activation, which creates the preconditions for the development of hyperpigmentation. Inflammation further increases the risk of pigmentation. The use of depigmenting agents in "home" dosages, anti-inflammatory agents, and plant extracts that inhibit melanin synthesis, in combination with UV filters and antioxidants, reduces the risk of hyperpigmentation.

6. **Stimulation of skin renewal.** As wonderful as peels are, they are not a magical elixir that miraculously changes skin properties. Visible improvements occur because there are cells in the skin that can build new skin. The activation of these cells is the lever that triggers repair and structural rejuvenation. It's also apparent that you can only get rejuvenation effects in this way as long as the cells can build new skin. This means that regeneration is impossible if these cells are damaged or depleted.

The result of any peeling is determined not only by how deeply we manage to damage the skin but also by how well we activate the remodeling processes. Incorporating remodeling activators into your home care can significantly enhance the effect of any peel.

Home treatments to stimulate remodeling include retinoids, vitamin C, remodeling peptides, and plant extracts that can stimulate collagen synthesis, such as centella or brown seaweed extracts.

The concentration of vitamin A and its esters depends on the purpose of the cosmetic product (**Table III-1-3**), as well as on its objectives. Care preparations are used on a permanent basis and are intended for the physiological regulation of skin cells in order to prevent/treat signs of aging, photoaging, and sebum secretion activity. Peel preparations are single-acting agents aimed at stimulating intensive exfoliation.

In preventive preparations, vitamin A and its ester concentrations are usually below average. Products for treating the signs of photodamage have higher concentrations. The highest concentration of retinol (about 1%) is found in products for intensive rejuvenation, which are essentially peeling products (see Part II, section 2.1.8).

Sometimes several forms of vitamin A are included in the formulation, for example:

- retinol esters + retinol
- retinol esters + retinol + retinal

These inactive precursors are at different stages of retinoic acid bio-synthesis (see **Fig. III-1-8**) and are, therefore, activated at different rates. Using such combinations makes it possible to increase the total concentration of vitamin A in the cosmetic product and ensure its gradual activation, thereby prolonging the product action while maintaining its safety.

It is also important to understand that collagen and elastin synthesis alone does not guarantee that the skin will look smooth and fresh. All these proteins must also be organized in the right way. However, the older the skin, the greater the risk that it lacks important regulators necessary for properly organizing collagen–elastin fibers. One such regulator is protein decorin. Cosmetic products may contain its synthetic analogue — tetrapeptide decorinil, which affects collagen synthesis similarly to decorin. The copper-containing peptide GHK-Cu may also be added to stimulate the synthesis of the skin's own decorin.

In-home care also depends on the purpose of the peel. For example, home care will include products that address these specific problems in the case of acne or post-acne skin.

For dark ethnic skin, in-home care includes depigmenting agents, anti-inflammatory substances, and antioxidants.

Sun protection should not be forgotten either. Products with UV filters should be used when the skin barrier is restored. Until then, avoiding sun exposure is the best and safest protection.

1.2.2. After the depigmenting treatment

An in-salon professional depigmenting procedure is only a part of skin lightening therapy. Without in-home care, the procedure's intended effect may fail to materialize or be minimal and short-lived. Therefore, the impact of lightening products should not be interrupted, as the pigment synthesis will otherwise soon return to its previous level. All these products were listed in the intensive exposure section — the difference will be in the doses (see Part III, chapter 4).

For dark ethnic skin, you can expect it to actively resist depigmenting, which can entail a paradoxical increase in pigmentation. Without well-designed in-home care, all efforts to lighten the skin will go to waste.

After the procedure, anti-inflammatory, antioxidant, and exfoliating agents need to be included in the in-home care regimen, along with substances that inhibit melanogenesis, such as arbutin, and extracts of licorice, mulberry, bearberry, and aloe. The skin must be carefully protected from the sun.

1.3. In-home skincare routine is key to the success of any aesthetic treatment

It would be great if a beautician had a magic wand that instantly solved all problems. However, like any biological system, skin cannot change immediately. Intense treatment only triggers specific processes, which then develop according to their own laws. Even the most advanced and highly active preparations won't have the desired effect without the active participation of the skin cells. This means that if we pin all our hopes on intensive action while neglecting the in-home care, we have as much chance of success as the team whose coach doesn't give enough time for regular training. No matter how inspirational a speech he gives before a match and how hard he tries to boost morale, the team will not have the resources to win.

By creating optimal conditions for skin cell function, by preventing or suppressing processes that could lead to undesirable effects such as severe inflammation, excessive pigmentation, or excessive destruction of intercellular lipid structures, and by supporting and stimulating regeneration processes, in-home care products greatly enhance the effectiveness of all treatments, and contribute to the development of a skincare culture in the consumer.

In-home care, including both preparation for procedures and rehabilitation after them, should not be the cherry on the cake but an indispensable link in comprehensive cosmetic care programs. Today, all professional cosmetic lines have products for in-home care. Unlike mass-market products, professional home remedies usually have a higher concentration of active ingredients and are formulated to the skin's needs before and after specific cosmetic procedures.

In general, daily in-home care includes the basic steps of intensive care but with the use of less concentrated and less aggressive agents (see Part IV, section 1.1):

- Cleansing
- Using active cosmetic products (serums, creams, masks) for specific aesthetic problems
- Strengthening the skin's barrier structures and moisturizing
- Maintaining a healthy microbiome
- Protection from the sun and external factors

1.4. Eye skincare

Eye skincare raises many questions, starting with whether skin products can be used to care for this area. To answer this and other questions, we need to look at the anatomy.

1.4.1. Eyelid skin peculiarities

The eyelid skin has a unique structure because the eyelids have a special function — they protect the eyeball from bright light, wind, and small particles. In addition, the eyelids help create and maintain a moist environment, which is necessary to prevent the cornea from drying out — during blinking, the borders of the eyelids are in contact, which allows moisture (tear film) to be redistributed over its surface. For the eyelids to perform all these functions, they need to "show" extreme softness and flexibility, which is why they are constructed in such a special way.

The eyelids generally consist of two layers: anterior (dermal-muscular) and posterior (mucociliary-cartilaginous). They have their own features, but the most important difference for the skin is that it is **very thin** — the thinnest on the whole body (Shriner D.L., Maibach H.I., 1996). Although the thickness of the entire epidermis on the eyelids is relatively normal, the thickness of the *stratum corneum* and dermis is the smallest — the thinnest area is on the inner (medial) side of the upper eyelid. Moreover, the subcutaneous layer contains almost no fatty tissue (Chopra K. et al., 2015). It turns out that the muscular layer (the circular muscle of the eye) adjoins almost close to the skin itself. Moreover, wrinkles are formed much easier in the periorbital area — not only is this area very mobile, but the extremely thin dermal layer cannot compensate for creases. The possibility of such mobility is provided by active innervation and blood supply.

Usually, the large size of corneocytes indicates a slow renewal of the epidermis. On the one hand, this allows keratinocytes to "mature" and effectively perform their functions on the skin surface (Grove G.L., Kligman A.M., 1983). On the other hand, the number of cell layers in the *stratum corneum* within the eyelid area is smaller than on other parts of the face, so even mature corneocytes cannot form a sufficiently strong barrier. As a result, the *stratum corneum* of the eyelid skin is not able to perform the barrier function as well as in the neighboring skin areas (Pratchyapruit W. et al., 2007). At the same time, the activity of sebaceous glands is also reduced, which leads to a lack of hydrolipid mantle (pH on the eyelids is more alkaline than in the adjacent areas) — this further reduces the effectiveness of the barrier (Zlotogorski A., 1987). Consequently, the eyelid skin is characterized by dryness and hypersensitivity, which may occur much earlier than age-related dryness and sensitivity of the facial skin.

It is interesting, as noted above, that the thickness of the eyelid epidermis is comparable to that in the neighboring areas, although its cell layers may be less developed. This is also due to the increased number of glycosaminoglycans in the intercellular space of the epidermis — as we know, they (in particular, the most striking representative — hyaluronic acid) can bind water.

The increased number of glycosaminoglycans, the branched blood supply system, and the thinness of eyelid skin explain the easy occurrence of **eyelid edema** in both local and systemic processes.

That presents the answer to the question posed at the beginning of this section — can facial products be used in the periorbital area? No, it is undesirable because many facial care products contain hygroscopic components, which provoke puffiness. Moreover, specialized eye products can also provoke puffiness and sensitivity, so their selection is not simple.

1.4.2. Problems in the periorbital area

Before moving on to recommendations for choosing eyelid skincare products, let's summarize the most common problems in this area:

- **Swollen eyelids** and **bags under the eyes** (it is important to determine the cause and identify renal, cardiac, allergic, anemia, rheumatism, myxedema, or menopause-related edema)

- **Dryness** and **scaling of the eyelid skin**
- **Hypersensitivity of the eyelid skin**
- **Dark circles around the eyes** can be caused by translucent blood vessels (blue or burgundy tint) or pigmentation (brown tint). Pigmentation can be caused by a reaction to UV radiation, post-inflammatory phenomena, or by systemic conditions such as atopic dermatitis, pregnancy chloasma, thyrotoxicosis, chrysoderma, etc.
- **Multiple wrinkles.** It is important to note that wrinkles around the eyes (including "crow's feet") can appear fairly early due to impaired visual acuity because the patient is squinting. In this situation, a consultation with an ophthalmologist is recommended. The examination by an ophthalmologist for rapid skin changes in the periorbital area is advised in any case because many processes in this area can be triggered by visual impairment and eye diseases.

Also, over time, there is an age-related loss of tissue volume under the eyes due to the downward displacement of facial fat packs. However, this problem, as well as the problem of upper and lower eyelid hernia formation and the zygomatic area, cannot be solved by cosmetic means — injectable, physical, and surgical methods are used for this purpose. Therefore, below we focus only on the above problems. It is important to note that these problems are rarely isolated. Usually, several are present at the same time.

Some of the external factors that provoke the mentioned problems include the effect of UV radiation, smoking, active makeup, and eyelash extensions — in the superimposed way (it makes the act of blinking less effective, plus lashes are attached using a special glue that can irritate tissues) or with the help of eyelash growth stimulants (active pharmaceutical agents used for this purpose can provoke inflammation).

1.4.3. Caring for the periorbital skin

As we explained above, **using products specifically designed for eye skincare is important**. They must pass an ophthalmological control and preferably contain no potential allergens: dyes, fragrances, or essential oils.

An important point: the pH of the finished product for eyelid skincare should be about 7.0–7.2, i.e., about the same pH as tears, so as not to irritate the eyes when the product gets on the lash.

For **cleansing**, it is recommended to use products with mild surfactants. More active surfactants can be used as needed (e.g., to remove makeup), but they must rinse off well. Two-phase cleansers can also be used for the eye area.

As **a basic care**, it is recommended to use gels, and lamellar emulsions — products with a light texture that contain **physiological lipids** — phospholipids (lecithin), ceramides, and cholesterol. Products that include **hygroscopic agents** (moisture catchers) — hyaluronic acid, collagen, glycerin — can be used **with extreme caution**, and if swelling occurs, their use must be immediately discontinued. Care must also be taken when using oils with a predominance of saturated fatty acids — they should be applied only in cases of pronounced skin dryness.

As for the active ingredients, their choice (and hence the choice of a particular product) will depend on the patient's existing problems.

- **Puffiness, dark "vascular" circles under the eyes** (to stimulate microcirculation) — caffeine, niacinamide, horse chestnut extract, green tea extract, aescin, centella extract, cornflower extract, vitamin C
- **Pigmentation** — caffeine, niacinamide, vitamin C, alpha-arbutin, tranexamic acid, resveratrol, licorice extract, lactic acid, brightening peptides, etc.
- **Laxity and wrinkles** — vitamin C, vitamin E, remodeling and neuromodulator peptides, plant stem cells, resveratrol, niacinamide, jojoba oil, shea butter, macadamia oil, evening primrose oil, retinol in low concentration and ester form (not recommended for sensitive skin)

It is also desirable for the product to contain **pro-** and **prebiotics** to maintain a healthy microbiome.

It is necessary to **protect the eyelid skin from ultraviolet light**. However, typical sunscreens have a rather thick consistency and occlusive properties, so they are uncomfortable and can provoke swelling. Because of this, sunglasses are the recommended method for protecting the periorbital area from the sun, and the cream should only be applied if it is impossible to wear them. To even out the negative UV effects, products should also contain antioxidants.

1.5. Lip care

The most common lip problems are dryness, scaling, and cracking due to the peculiarities of the skin structure consisting of three parts: the perioral skin, lips, and mucosa.

- The **perioral skin**, like the skin of the face, has appendages (glands and hair follicles). However, its dermal layer is thinner, the fat layer is almost absent, and the muscle layer is very pronounced. Therefore, early mimic wrinkles (facial expression lines) are formed here.
- The **skin of the lips**, with three to five cell layers, is very thin compared to typical facial skin, which has up to 16 layers. With light skin color, the lip skin contains fewer melanocytes. Because of this, the blood vessels are visible, which leads to the notable red coloring. With darker skin color, this effect is less prominent, as in this case the skin of the lips contains more melanin and thus is visually darker. The lip skin forms the border between the exterior skin of the face and the interior mucous membrane of the oral cavity. The lip skin is not hairy and does not have sebaceous and sweat glands, that is why it is not covered by a natural hydrolipid protective layer, which keeps the skin smooth and mild, suppresses pathogens, and regulates TEWL (Arai S. et al., 1989). For these reasons, the lips dry out faster and become chapped more easily.
- The **mucous membrane** occupies the back surface of the lips and is covered by a multi-layered squamous, non-keratinized epithelium. The secretion of the lip salivary glands wets it. The mucous membrane is represented by a large area in the sensory cortex of the central nervous system and is, therefore, highly sensitive.

The lip epidermis renews itself very quickly and has no time to mature (Arai S. et al., 1990). As a result, corneocytes and intercellular lipid layers do not form a sufficiently dense barrier. The lip epidermis remains more permeable than the barrier of normal skin, leading to accelerated water loss and dryness. In addition, the latter provokes another problem. It is believed that the degradation of desmosomes providing adhesion of epidermal cells plays a role in trypsin and chymotrypsin-like enzymes, and the water content of the *stratum corneum* is mentioned as a factor regulating the activity of these enzymes. Accordingly, if it is lacking, the enzymes do not work efficiently enough, and full-fledged destruction of desmosomes does not occur — as a result, we see scaling (Hikima R. et al., 2004). It is aggravated by various external factors — cold temperatures, sharp temperature contrasts, wind, UV exposure, and dry air in heated rooms in winter — since under these conditions of insufficient barrier skin functions, more water is lost, and desquamation processes are disturbed even more. In addition, against the background of dryness, some cracks cause significant discomfort — as mentioned above, the skin of the lips is very actively innervated.

Accordingly, balms containing occlusive components, i.e., those that prevent water evaporation from the skin, are considered the main lip care product.

As we know, there are two fundamentally different ways to moisturize the *stratum corneum*. The first is to use a non-aqueous ointment based on Vaseline or silicone, which creates an occlusive layer on the skin to inhibit water evaporation: water accumulates in the *stratum corneum*, and its hydration level increases.

The second way is to introduce water from outside with the help of water-rich preparations. These can be gels (water + colloid) or emulsions (water + oil), which contain components that bind water (moisturizing agents). Low-molecular-weight moisturizing agents (such as NMF components and ions) penetrate the *stratum corneum*, accumulate in it, and attract water. High-molecular-weight compounds (proteins, polysaccharides, glycols) remain on the skin surface, forming a wet compress.

In lip care products, petroleum jelly is often the main ingredient, as it is considered one of the strongest occlusive agents. However, it only retains moisture without restoring the natural barrier properties of the lips. In fact, it has the opposite effect — because petroleum jelly is too moisturizing, it can slow down the restoration of the epidermal barrier, and the cells do not get the signal in time that the barrier needs to be repaired.

It is generally believed that occlusive products are necessary for permanent use if barrier function cannot be restored (e.g., in atopic dermatitis due to genetic defects). However, when you stop using them, things usually go back to normal. Some people even develop a kind of addiction to lip balms — if they apply them, there is a relief, but as soon as they stop using them, dryness and flaking return. Therefore, if there is still a chance to restore barrier structures, occlusive products should be used only for the initial phase.

In the case of the barrier function of the lips, there is such a chance. Restoring the skin's natural protective barrier is another way to increase skin hydration. Recent studies have shown that, in the lipid layers of the *stratum corneum*, there is an imbalance of ceramides — one of the main (and most significant in quantity) components of the lipid barrier along with cholesterol and free fatty acids (all these lipids are referred to the so-called physiological lipids) (Ishikawa J. et al., 2013; Shimotoyodome Y. et al., 2014). Intercellular lipids of the *stratum corneum* bind ("cement") the scales together and form the basis of the permeability barrier (lipid barrier), which prevents the diffusion of substances through the *stratum corneum* in both directions. A change in the ratio of lipids in the lipid barrier leads to the impairment of its function.

It has been revealed that in the lips' *stratum corneum*, the amount of ceramides per se is reduced, while their imbalance is also observed — a higher percentage of ceramide subtypes such as Cer [NS] (with short-chain Cer [NS] dominating) and Cer [AS], and a lower percentage of Cer [NP] and Cer [NH] compared to other skin areas of the body (Ishikawa J. et al., 2013; Shimotoyodome Y. et al., 2014).

In a recent study, Japanese scientists investigated whether ceramides reduce lip dryness and flakiness as effectively as highly occlusive formulations. They used a synthetic pseudoceramide (pCer; INCI: Cetyl-PG Hydroxyethyl Palmitamide) that was already proven effective in treating atopic dermatitis. Moreover, this pseudoceramide was included in a product that does not provide occlusion.

Thirty-one healthy women (aged 21 to 37; mean age 28.6 years) with normal skin and dry lips participated. The women were divided into three groups according to the product used: a control (a ceramide-free product with moderate occlusive properties), a non-occlusive product with 0.5% pCer, and a product with 2.0% pCer. Each product was applied four times daily (morning, noon, evening, and bedtime) for four weeks. The degrees of lip roughness, lip moisture, TEWL rate, and lip surface elasticity were assessed. Endogenous ceramide profiles and the level of pCer absorption in the *stratum corneum* were also determined (Tamura E. et al., 2020; Tamura E. et al., 2021).

After four weeks, the group of women who used 2.0% pCer showed a significant reduction in roughness compared to the initial level and to the group that used preparation with a lower ceramide concentration as well as women that used the occlusive control agent. Moreover, the improvement increased by Week 4, whereas the effect of the 0.5% agent only became apparent by that time. By Week 4, the 2.0% pCer group also showed a decrease in TEWL, along with an increase in moisturization and lip elasticity. Interestingly, moisturization and TEWL rates also improved in the group using the occlusive control agent by Week 2 but then gradually decreased. There was also a decrease in the amount of Cer [NS], an increased concentration of which is found not only on the lips but also in atopic dermatitis, i.e., it is a marker of skin barrier failure (Imokawa G., 2009). The amount of Cer [NH], the low content of which has a high correlation with lip roughness, and Cer [NP] also increased.

As for the absorption of pCer, it is quite natural that its higher content leads to better absorption. In addition, absorption can also be affected by the condition of the skin: the rougher it is, the higher the absorption.

What conclusions can be drawn from this information? For lip care, it is effective to use not just occlusive products that retain water but to strengthen the natural barrier function of the lip skin with physiological lipids in the form of primarily ceramides. The better the lipid barrier is restored, the less reliance is placed on classic Vaseline-based lip balms.

1.6. Hand skincare

Although this book does not deal with body care (see the *Body Contouring in Cosmetic Dermatology & Skincare Practice* book), we do want to talk about the care for the skin on the hands. Hands are more exposed than other body parts and even the face to mechanical stress, contact with chemicals, temperature fluctuations, and sun exposure. Even if the skin of the hands is healthy, improper care can cause dryness and

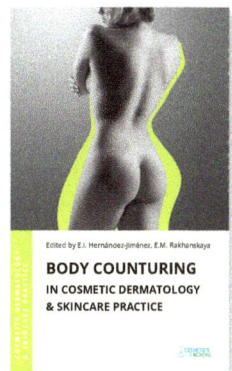

Edited by E.I. Hernández-Jiménez, E.M. Rakhanskaya

BODY CONTURING
IN COSMETIC DERMATOLOGY
& SKINCARE PRACTICE

tightness, small wrinkles, and cracks. It's well-known that the hand skin ages faster than the rest of the body. However, everyone wants to see their hands young, well-groomed, and attractive. To achieve this, three barriers must be taken care of:

1) microbial
2) epidermal
3) immune

Before moving on to exactly how this can be achieved, let's briefly review the features specific to hand skin.

1.6.1. Peculiarities of the hand skin structure

Numerous folds and small joints on the hands facilitate complex movements: touching, stroking, hitting, scratching, and holding. That is why the **palm skin** is quite thick — in its epidermis, there is the pronounced *stratum lucidum* between the *stratum granulosum* and *stratum corneum*. There are many sweat glands on the palms and no hair follicles at all. The fingertips have high sensitivity, which is provided by a large number of nerve endings. The **skin of the back of the hands** is thin and elastic. It has weak subcutaneous fatty tissue. There are few (but there are) hair follicles and sweat glands in this area.

Thus, the physiological features of hand skin include **the ability to increase sweating, increased motor activity and sensitivity, and excellent regeneration capabilities**.

We should also not forget to mention the **hydrolipid (acidic) mantle** that covers the skin of the hands. Its components are the secretions of sweat and sebaceous glands, exfoliated epidermis, and small amounts of epidermal lipids. When mixed, they form an emulsion consisting of aqueous and fatty phases with a slightly acidic (but one of the highest on the body) pH of 5–5.5. The hydrolipid mantle is home to the entire skin microbiome, and its stable acidity prevents pathogenic bacteria from multiplying. It provides softness, elasticity, and absence of cracks on the skin, which protects the *stratum corneum*, the skin's main barrier structure.

Corneocytes and intercellular substances provide the unique structure of the *stratum corneum*. Corneocytes are tightly adjoining cells filled with keratin, surrounded by a lipid-protein cornified envelope and interconnected by corneodesmosomes. Between the cells are intercellular lipids organized into lipid bilayers and represented mainly by ceramides, cholesterol, and fatty acids. This structure of the *stratum corneum* of the epidermis prevents pathogenic substances from entering the epidermis and prevents excessive TEWL.

In addition, the epidermis provides immune protection due to the **Langerhans cells** in it, which are capable of movement. They recognize who is "ours" and who is "alien" among those substances that have managed to pass through the *stratum corneum*. Langerhans cells are innate immunity carriers — often the starting point of allergic reactions and inflammatory processes.

1.6.2. Hand skin microbiome

As mentioned above, maintaining healthy and youthful hand skin involves maintaining its three barriers: microbial, epidermal, and immune. In terms of the microbial barrier, there are many microorganisms living on hands that belong to four phyla (phylum is a taxonomic category above a class but below a kingdom) (**Fig. V-1-1**) (Edmonds-Wilson S.L. et al., 2015):

1. Actinobacteria — *Mycobacteriaceae spp.*, *Streptomyces spp.*
2. Proteobacteria — *Enterobacteriaceae spp.*, *Pseudomonas aeruginosa*, *Escherichia coli*, *Helicobacter pylori*, etc.
3. Firmicutes — *Staphylococcus aureus*, *Clostridium botulinum*, *Lactobacillus spp.*
4. Bacteroidetes

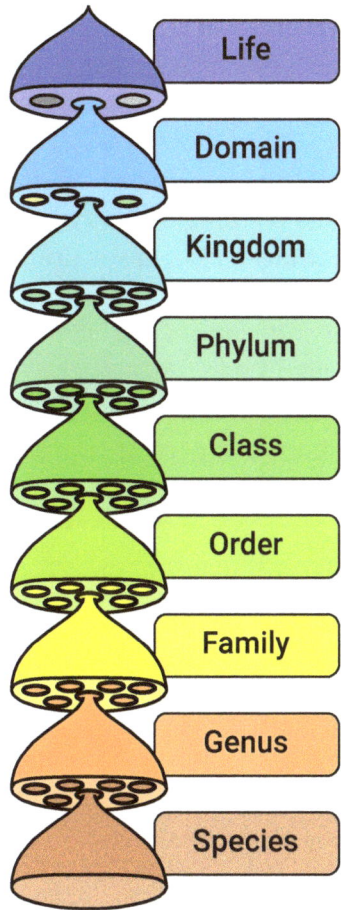

Figure V-1-1. Hierarchy of major taxonomic ranks in biology

All microorganisms on the skin can be divided into those that are present permanently (**resident microflora**) and temporarily (**transient microflora**). They are usually found in the upper layers of the epidermis, which are in contact with the environment, in the mouths of sweat glands, greasy hair follicles, and in the acid (hydrolipid) mantle of the skin. The microbial composition of men's and women's hands differs significantly, as do the hands of people of different professions and lifestyles.

The hand microbiome is generally more diverse than in other parts of the body because the hands are constantly in contact with many "alien" microorganisms. The palms and forearms are the richest in this respect, while the back of the hands is the poorest (Vandegrift R. et al., 2017). Resident microflora is more resistant to external influences and is challenging to eliminate, while transient microflora easily leaves the hand skin.

The microbiome's composition is influenced by a person's sex, environment, place of residence, hygiene habits, and presence of pets (Vandegrift R. et al., 2017). The risk of hand contamination with pathogens increases dramatically when visiting the toilet (especially during diarrhea), changing diapers of a sick child, blowing the nose, and in contact with raw food (Todd E.C.D. et al., 2010). Interestingly, microorganisms living on the hands during desquamation of corneocytes can also disperse into the air, creating a personal "microbial cloud" of a person or animal (Vandegrift R. et al., 2017).

The microbial profile constantly changes due to constant exfoliation of corneocyte epidermal cells, contact with various objects, washing the skin, and applying creams. Not all microorganisms are harmful — there are conditionally "good" (saprophytes) and "bad" (pathogens) microorganisms. It is important that **normally they are in a ratio that does not allow infectious diseases to develop and the hands remain healthy**.

Therefore, maintaining a balanced microbial association is essential for skin health. In this regard, the previously strongly promoted concept of hand hygiene to eliminate all microflora is now under serious reconsideration.

1.6.3. Impact of hand washing on the microbiome

Any detergent affects the entire microbial composition of the skin — it does not care which bacteria are "good" or "bad." As a result, the total number of bacteria is reduced, and if the detergent contains antiseptics, it is reduced significantly. However, no cleaning method (including ethanol and sanitizers) leads to the complete elimination of microflora (Zapka C. et al., 2017).

After washing and antiseptic treatment, the microbial association is gradually replenished by bacteria from other areas of the skin and from other people, the air, and objects. It is most actively replenished by the microflora left on the skin (in folds, under the nail plate, and cuticle). Will the microbiome's composition be the same as before the hygiene treatment? Most likely yes, if you washed your hands at home, and no, if you went to a hospital, clinic, beauty parlor, workplace, or public restroom.

Does this mean that we risk bacterial infection when we wash our hands, getting the opposite of the desired effect? It depends on the technique and frequency of hand washing, the detergent, and the condition of the skin's barrier function.

1.6.4. Hand washing technique

Teaching proper handwashing is a big problem (Smith W.P. et al., 2007). There is a European standard for handwashing EN1500, which describes the sequence of movements.

According to this standard, each of the six movements is repeated five times, and the entire treatment takes about 1 min (**Fig. V-1-2**). The water should be slightly warm, and the detergent should only be applied to wet hands. Rings and other jewelry should always be removed. It is important to rub hands together thoroughly during washing, wiping the skin in folds and around the nails. **The faucet is closed with the towel with which you wipe your hands.**

1.6.5. Frequency of hand washing

Even if your job doesn't require you to always wash your hands, you probably do it twice a day, morning and evening. In addition, you probably wash your hands before you eat (and sometimes after you eat) and after you go to the bathroom and take a shower, which adds up to 5–7 times a day. You can add another 15–20 times to the total

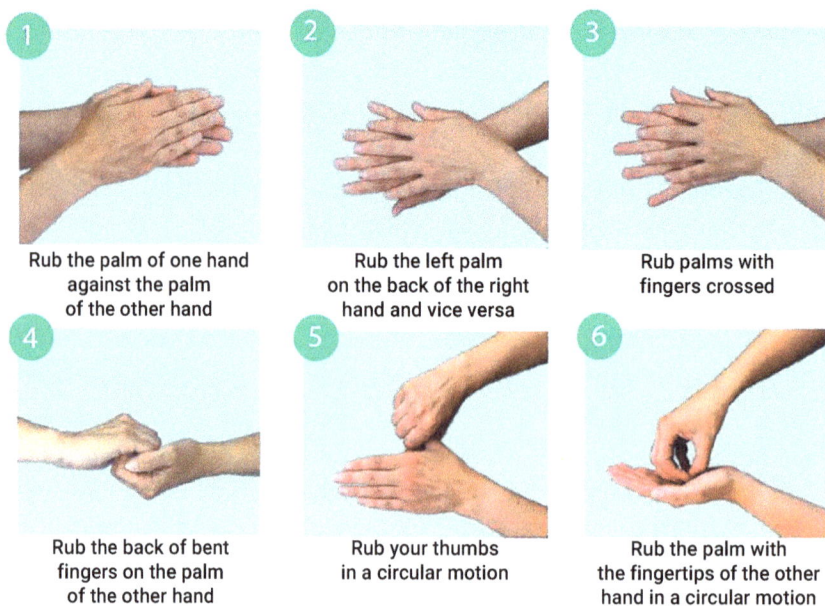

1 Rub the palm of one hand against the palm of the other hand	**2** Rub the left palm on the back of the right hand and vice versa	**3** Rub palms with fingers crossed
4 Rub the back of bent fingers on the palm of the other hand	**5** Rub your thumbs in a circular motion	**6** Rub the palm with the fingertips of the other hand in a circular motion

Figure V-1-2. The sequence of handwashing steps according to the European Hand Washing Standard EN1500

if you're a medic. With the arrival of the coronavirus pandemic, almost everyone had to become "medics" (according to the intensity of hand washing).

But even in the pre-COVID era, according to published World Health Organization (WHO) data, out of every 100 patients hospitalized, at least 7 in developed countries and 10 in developing countries acquired healthcare-associated infections (WHO, 2013). WHO has developed a *Clean Care is Safer Care* program for workers who come in contact with sick people. It describes the five main points at which it is important for a healthcare professional to wash their hands:

1) before touching the patient
2) before aseptic procedures (including catheter placement)
3) after contact with any biological fluids
4) after contact with the patient's body
5) after contact with the patient's belongings

Can the epidermal barrier take such strain? Water, especially chlorinated and hot water, dries out the skin even without detergent, degrading its barrier properties. **Hence, you should wash your hands with slightly warm water and do it relatively quickly.**

1.6.6. Hand detergents

Detergents and disinfectants contribute to the disruption of the epidermal barrier. Almost all chunky soaps, including baby soaps, have an alkaline pH and shift the weakly acidic pH of the skin to the alkaline side during washing (Barrett-Hill F., 2009). This leads to changes in the microbiome, promoting the multiplication of pathogenic microorganisms.

A paradox arises: frequent hand washing increases the number of germs due to the deterioration of skin health (Larson E., 1999). Therefore, it is better to use syndet detergents (liquid soaps with added conditioners — oils or creams) with a neutral or slightly acidic pH designed for hand washing while rinsing the detergent thoroughly. Antibacterial additives for routine hand washing (even in medical practice) are unnecessary and undesirable. Surfactants in detergents can destroy the shells of bacteria and viruses themselves. There is no additional need for antibiotics in detergents.

1.6.7. Hand drying

The speed of the process itself measures the effectiveness of hand drying, the final dryness of the skin, the elimination of bacteria, and the prevention of cross-contamination (Huang C. et al., 2012). What options are available in this area? Hands can be dried with a regular waffle or terry towel, paper towels, a simple electric dryer, or a non-contact instant dryer (**Fig. V-1-3**).

The achievable dryness of the skin varies:

- after using the towel, 4% moisture remains on the skin

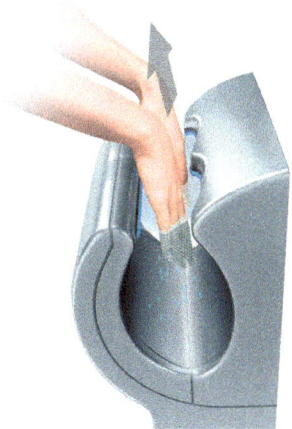

Figure V-1-3. Instant dryer operating principle: air flow, like a blade, shaves water off hands

- after a conventional electric dryer — 3% moisture
- after paper towel and contactless dryer — 1% moisture

The speed of drying hands with hot air in a conventional dryer is at least 40 seconds; with a towel and instant dryer, about 10 seconds. Studies have shown that both women and men spend far less time drying their hands than necessary. As a result, hands remain wet and microbial contamination of the skin increases (Patrick D. et al., 1997).

In terms of cleanliness, wiping your hands with a cloth towel is the least hygienic option, suitable only for the home. It is better to wipe your hands with a paper towel, but bacteria from the air can be deposited on the paper. In addition, if the dispenser uses recycled paper, it can retain resistant strains of microorganisms. A conventional electric dryer's filter is contaminated over time by bacteria that concentrate in the ambient air. These bacteria can settle on clothing and skin and enter the respiratory tract. Moreover, under the influence of hot air, the skin becomes dry and rough, i.e., the epidermal barrier is violated. In this regard, the instant hand dryer is the best option because it does not come into contact with the hands, dries them with slightly warm air, and is equipped with an antibacterial filter (Mutters R. et al., 2019). But it is also the most expensive.

A very important factor in hand cleansing is hand friction, both when washing and when drying. When rubbing on the towel, microorganisms escape from the skin folds, hair follicle mouths, and sweat glands and remain on the towel. When drying with hot air, rubbing hands against each other also helps release germs, which are either distributed to neighboring skin areas or released into the surrounding air. So from this point of view, wiping with a paper towel is preferable (Huang C. et al., 2012).

Does the quality of the paper matter? Yes, it does because it determines its absorbency. Also, stiff paper scratches your hands and doesn't dry them effectively.

Does it matter how the paper is fed? Yes, an open container paper roll is the worst because germs from the air are easily deposited on the paper. A roll in a closed container or, even better, one with a dispenser is a better option.

1.6.8. After-cleansing recovery

Frequent exposure to water and detergents damages the epidermal barrier. Applying a moisturizing cream can help restore its function — it is recommended to do this after each hand wash. The cream is distributed on the skin by capturing interdigital spaces and cuticle until completely absorbed.

Many people think it is better to use baby cream or apply the same cream to all body parts, and the most economical apply the rest of the face cream on their hands. This is wrong. Hand cream should not be greasy, even if the skin is dry. The skin under a layer of cream should dry, not sweat. The presence of occlusive substances in such skincare products is undesirable.

The cream must absorb well and quickly so as not to interfere with the subsequent work. This property depends on its hydrophilicity (usually the water content is 70–90%), as well as on the humidity and temperature of the ambient air. The exact duration of cream absorption has not been established, but on average it is about one minute (Hines J. et al., 2017).

The amount of cream also matters, so a bottle with a dispenser is preferable to a standard tube — when you press it, it gives a standard dose, no more or less. It is important that the cream rinses off well because it washes off the substances and germs that get on the skin.

Additionally, applying the cream in the morning and at night is recommended. The morning application helps rinse harmful substances from the skin easily, and the night application provides long-lasting restoration of the epidermal barrier. But these should be different creams: a protective cream in the morning and a nourishing cream in the evening.

Protective cream

The protective cream is designed to protect the skin of the hands against the adverse effects of environmental factors (e.g., detergents, aggressive liquids, oils, wind). It is applied immediately before contact with aggressive factors. Usually, this cream is poorly absorbed into the skin, so it takes longer than usual to apply it.

The cream's silicone, glycerin, waxes, and mineral oils form an enveloping film, a kind of "invisible gloves." They protect the skin from drying, irritation, and peeling. And as these "gloves" have to work, they have special requirements: they must not be slippery, cause increased sweating, leave greasy imprints on objects, and be easy to wash off.

Professional protective creams can be hydrophilic (for working with technical oils, petroleum products, paint, fiberglass, and other water-insoluble substances), hydrophobic (for working with acids, bases, lime, cement, fertilizers, detergents and disinfectants, and other water-soluble substances) and combined.

Nourishing cream

The main purpose of nourishing hand creams is to restore the epidermal barrier in general and the hydrolipid mantle of the skin in particular. Nourishing creams include substances that eliminate dryness, soften rough skin, have an anti-inflammatory and healing effect, and improve microcirculation. As a rule, these are vegetable oils, vitamins, antioxidants, urea, and herbal extracts.

Nourishing creams are greasier than moisturizers and take longer to absorb. They are best applied at night or after housework and evening showers when no more contact with water is expected.

Today, there are many hand creams with dual effect — moisturizing and nourishing — on the market.

1.6.9. Preventing inflammatory diseases

Frequent hand washing, prolonged contact with water, and prolonged wear of gloves are unavoidable in many professions. Doctors, nurses, nurse practitioners, skincare specialists, hairdressers, food industry workers, and cooks are constantly faced with this issue (Smith S., 2009).

According to German Clinical Guidelines (www.baua.de), **wet work is defined as work in which the hands are wet or in occlusive gloves for more than two hours per shift or if the hands are washed more than 20 times a day**. These people are at an increased risk for developing contact dermatitis and eczema. In many organizations, it is mandatory to apply protective cream before starting work (reduces the penetration of irritants into the skin, supports the skin's own protection, makes it easier to wash away dirt), and moisturizing cream after each hand wash and at the end of work. An appropriate container with a dispenser is attached near the sink, along with instructions for use.

Despite this increasingly common practice, the compliance of workers at risk remains rather low (Hines J. et al., 2017). The launch of the "Healthy Hands" project, which aims to change the attitudes of nurses and paramedics towards hand care products, has shown that the incidence of contact dermatitis and epidermal barrier disorders decreases if specific rules are followed (Soltanipoor M. et al., 2017). For several years now, tubes of moisturizing cream with a dispenser have been available in airline lavatories and hotels near sinks, reminding people to take care of their hands. This practice is now expanding. It would be ideal to have such devices in clinics, hospitals, and wherever there are at-risk employees.

Gloves should be worn when cleaning rooms, working with water and various liquids, and when in contact with vegetables, raw meat, and fish. Rubber, latex, or nitrile gloves are more suitable for fine work, and thick rubber gloves with a cotton lining inside are suitable for cleaning, washing, or dishwashing. Hands in gloves become moist quickly, and this environment is ideal for reproducing germs and fungi, especially candida.

To prevent skin diseases, gloves should be worn on clean, dry hands. If gloves are expected to be worn for more than five minutes, it is recommended to wear cotton gloves under them (Ibler K.S. et al., 2012). Even when such precautions are taken, hands sweat quickly. If this occurs, the gloves should be removed, hands should be dried, and a dry pair should be put on to continue working.

1.6.10. Hand care for contact dermatitis and eczema

Contact dermatitis and eczema are the most common inflammatory non-infectious hand diseases associated with a violation of the barrier properties of the epidermis. Among them, irritable (irritant) dermatitis, atopic contact dermatitis, and hand eczema can be distinguished etiologically (Veien N.K. et al., 2008; Mollerup A. et al., 2012). The average age of patients with irritable dermatitis is significantly lower than that of individuals affected by allergic dermatitis. The risk of contact dermatitis is increased for skincare practitioners, hairdressers, painters, cooks, butchers, bakers, and locksmiths (Schwensen J.F. et al., 2013). However, with the emergence of the SARS-CoV-2 pandemic in our lifetime, the risk of irritant dermatitis exists for al-

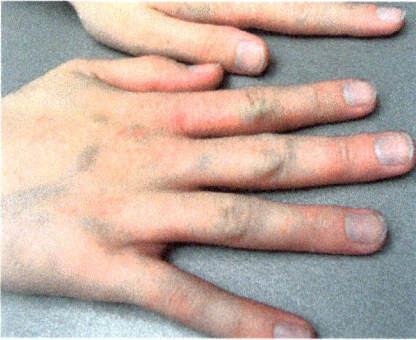

Figure V-1-4. Irritative dermatitis: rashes are seen in the interdigital spaces, which spread to the hand back (photo: Albanova V.I.)

most anyone. For this reason, we decided to devote a separate section to hand care for patients with dermatitis and eczema.

Irritant dermatitis is a dermatosis of the skin of the hands caused by prolonged contact with aggressive substances. Its acute stage is manifested by erythema, swelling, intensive scaling, and itching. In the long-term course, dryness, erythematous-squamous foci, cracks, and lichenification predominate. The rashes are often located in the interdigital spaces and may extend to the dorsal and palm surfaces of fingers and hands (**Fig. V-1-4**). Blisters are usually absent, itching is moderate, and burning, tingling, and pain may be present.

Atopic contact dermatitis occurs a few days after the first exposure to the allergen, and at repeated contact, it occurs immediately or within a few hours. Subjectively, it is characterized by pronounced itching with burning, tingling, and painful sensations. Clinically, it is characterized by blisters that merge, erythema, phlegm, and crusts. The most characteristic locations are the fingertips, the cuticle, and the back of the hands. Rashes may spread to the forearms (**Fig. V-1-5**). Hand lesions occur in about 60% of patients with atopic dermatitis (Golden S., Shaw T., 2013). It is common in adults and older children, and in adults, especially in women, it is often the only manifestation of the disease.

Eczema is caused by a combination of exogenous (aggressive contact substances, allergens) and endogenous factors (tendency to atopy, individual hypersensitivity). Regardless of the form of the disease, housewives and employees of medical institutions are more often affected by eczema of the hands. Exacerbations usually occur in the wintertime.

In one study, 67% of those surveyed reported that eczema impairs their personal life and negatively affects their daily activities (Park J.B. et al., 2016). In addition to the above signs characteristic of dermatitis, eczema presents with small clustered vesicles, erosions, and crusts. In the acute phase, small vesicles, erythema, and swelling predominate; in the chronic phase, infiltration, scaling, and cracking, often painful, predominate (**Fig. V-1-6**). According to German clinical Guidelines, eczema is considered chronic if it lasts more than three months and worsens at least twice a year (Diepgen T.L. et al., 2009).

In diagnosing all the above diseases, it helps to take a medical history. The most common localization of atopic dermatitis is the back of the hands and fingers. Erythematous-squamous plaques of pink color with indistinct boundaries, lichenification, dry skin, and itching are characteristic. Papules

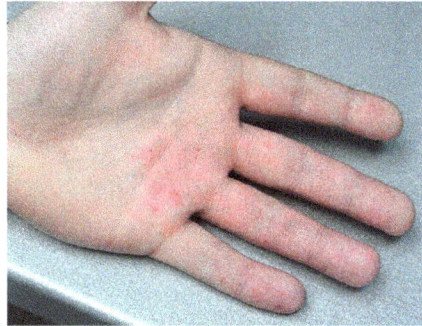

Figure V-1-5. Allergic contact dermatitis: affection of the tips and palm side of the fingers (erythema, small blisters, erosions, and crusts) is noted (photo: Albanova V.I.)

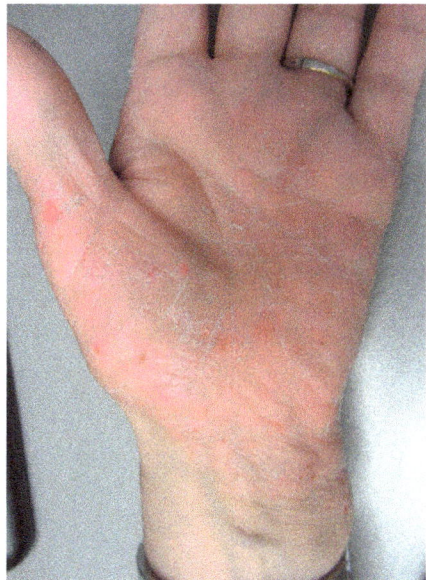

Figure V-1-6. Chronic hand eczema: infiltration, scaling, and skin cracks (photo: Albanova V.I.)

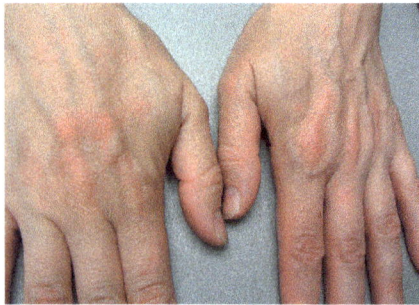

Figure V-1-7. Atopic hand eczema (photo: Albanova V.I.)

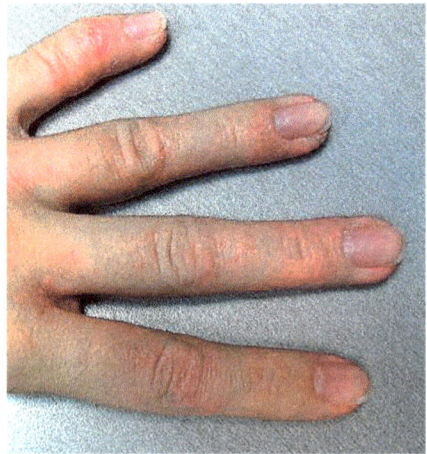

Figure V-1-8. Atopic hand eczema: edema of the cuticle, loss of the cuticle, changes in the shape of nails, erythematous-squamous focus on the little finger (photo: Albanova V.I.)

and vesicles may be present, especially during exacerbation of the disease (**Fig. V-1-7**). Skin rashes are accompanied by changes in the nails: loss of the cuticle, transverse furrows, and inflammation of the cuticle (**Fig. V-1-8**). These patients are often resistant to therapy. Combinations of atopic dermatitis with allergic rhinitis, pollinosis, and bronchial asthma are not uncommon.

Chronic nonatopic eczema has the same clinical manifestations as atopic eczema, but the dryness of the skin is milder in the former (**Fig. V-1-9**). It is often occupationally related and occurs in food workers, barbers, cosmetic aestheticians, construction workers, plumbers, and electricians. The most severe manifestations are noted in men, the elderly, and poorly educated people (Mollerup A. et al., 2012).

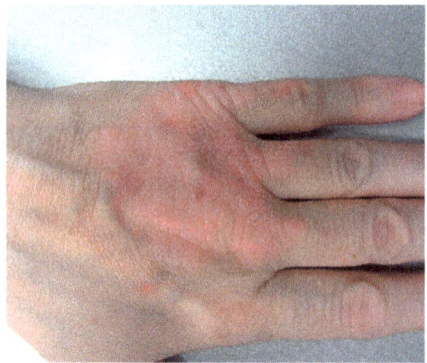

Figure V-1-9. Chronic non-atopic eczema (photo: Albanova V.I.)

Hand eczema accounts for 90% of all occupational skin diseases and ranks third among all occupational diseases in general. The magnitude of the problem is so great that a multidisciplinary approach to its solution is recommended: in addition to a dermatologist, the therapeutic team includes a care manager, a special nurse, and an occupational disease specialist (Van Gils R.F. et al., 2009).

Care recommendations

In the recent past, abstaining entirely from hand washing for eczema and dermatitis was recommended, as evidenced in old textbooks and manuals. This was good advice then since only coarse, lumpy soaps with a high pH were available. Unfortunately, to this day, many dermatologists still advise limiting hand washing. But how can a modern person with good hygiene habits give it up?

Professional advice for patients with eczema and dermatitis is as follows: use warm (not hot) water, sindet liquid hand soap, rinse well from the skin, and dry it thoroughly, then apply cream. It is better to use special hypoallergenic creams without fragrances with a minimum of auxiliary components.

Combination of moisturizers and topical medications

After washing and drying the hands, moisturizing cream should be applied, and after 15–20 minutes — the drug in the form of an ointment. If the drug is prescribed as a solution, emulsion, or cream, it should be applied first and the cream after 15–20 minutes.

The requirements for shower detergents are similar. After showering, moisturizing body cream is applied first (including on the hands), and the medication is applied after 15–20 minutes. Taking a bath, or going to the bathhouse, sauna, or swimming pool during the exacerbation of the inflammatory disease of the hands is undesirable.

To prevent and treat inflammatory diseases of the hands, it is nesessary to develop a skincare habit. It is important to know proper hand care — what and how to wash them, how to wipe them, and what cream to apply. Care is necessary for healthy and pathological hand skin — no fundamental differences exist. For workers at risk, it is advisable to have paper towels and moisturizing cream with a dispenser next to the sink in the workplace.

References

Anitha B. Prevention of complications in chemical peeling. J Cutan Aesthet Surg 2010; 3(3): 186–188.

Anju G. Tranexamic acid: An emerging depigmenting agent. Pigment International 2016; 3(2): 66–71.

Arai S., Oshida K., Hikima T., Fukuda Y. Study on lip surface-characteristics of stratum corneum and corneocytes on lip. J Jap Cosmet Sci Soc 1990; 14: 66–70.

Arai S., Oshida K., Hikima T., Hasunuma K. Study on lip surface-characteristics of chapped lip. J Jap Cosmet Sci Soc 1989; 13: 64–68.

Aßmus U., Banowski B., Brock M., et al. Impact of cleansing products on the skin surface pH. IFSCC Magazine 2013; 16: 17–24.

Barrett-Hill F. Cosmetic Chemistry. Virtual Beauty Corp., 2009.

Berson D. Recommendation of moisturizers and cleansers: a study of unmet needs among dermatology patients. Cutis 2005; 76(6 Suppl): 3–6.

Blanchet-Réthoré S., Bourdès V., Mercenier A., et al. Effect of a lotion containing the heat-treated probiotic strain Lactobacillus johnsonii NCC 533 on Staphylococcus aureus colonization in atopic dermatitis. Clin Cosmet Investig Dermatol 2017; 10: 249–257.

Boissy R.E., Visscher M., DeLong M.A. DeoxyArbutin: a novel reversible tyrosinase inhibitor with effective in vivo skin lightening potency. Exp Dermatol 2005; 14(8): 601–608.

Boonchai W., Iamtharachai P. The pH of commonly available soaps, liquid cleansers, detergents and alcohol gels. Dermatitis 2010; 21(3): 154–156.

Bos J.D., Meinardi M.M. The 500 Dalton rule for the skin penetration of chemical compounds and drugs. Exp Dermatol 2000; 9(3): 165–169.

Brocklehurst K., Philpott M.P. Cysteine proteases: mode of action and role in epidermal differentiation. Cell Tissue Res 2013; 351(2): 237–244.

Bruno B.J., Miller G.D., Lim C.S. Basics and recent advances in peptide and protein drug delivery. Ther Deliv 2013; 4(11): 1443–1467.

Bylka W., Znajdek-Awiżeń P., Studzińska-Sroka E., Brzezińska M. Centella asiatica in cosmetology. Postepy Dermatol Alergol 2013; 30(1): 46–49.

Callender V.D., St. Surin-Lord S., Davis E.C., Maclin M. Postinflammatory hyperpigmentation: etiologic and therapeutic considerations. Am J Clin Dermatol 2011; 12(2): 87–99.

Chaudhuri R.K., Bojanowski K. Bakuchiol: a retinol-like functional compound revealed by gene expression profiling and clinically proven to have anti-aging effects. Int J Cosmet Sci 2014; 36(3): 221–230.

Chhabra G., Garvey D.R., Singh C.K., et al. Effects and Mechanism of Nicotinamide Against UVA- and/or UVB-mediated DNA Damages in Normal Melanocytes. Photochem Photobiol 2019; 95(1): 331–337.

Cho Y.H., Park J.E., Lim D.S., Lee J.S. Tranexamic acid inhibits melanogenesis by activating the autophagy system in cultured melanoma cells. J Dermatol Sci 2017; 88(1): 96–102.

Choi J.E., Di Nardo A. Skin neurogenic inflammation. Seminars Immunopathol 2018; 40(3): 249–259.

Chopra K., Calva D., Sosin M., Tadisina K.K., Banda A., De La Cruz C., Chaudhry M.R., Legesse T., Drachenberg C.B., Manson P.N., Christy M.R. A comprehensive examination of topographic thickness of skin in the human face. Aesthet Surg J 2015; 35(8): 1007–1013.

Cohen J.L., Makino E., Sonti S., Mehta R. Synergistic combination of an In-office procedure and home regimen for the treatment of facial hyperpigmentation. J Clin Aesthet Dermatol 2012; 5(4): 33–35.

Davis E.C., Callender V.D. Postinflammatory hyperpigmentation: a review of the epidemiology, clinical features, and treatment options in skin of color. J Clin Aesthet Dermatol 2010; 3(7): 20–31.

Delinasios G.J., Karbaschi M., Cooke M.S., et al. Vitamin E inhibits the UVAI induction of «light» and «dark» cyclobutane pyrimidine dimers, and oxidatively generated DNA damage, in keratinocytes. Sci Rep 2018; 8(1): 423.

Dhaliwal S., Rybak I., Ellis S.R., et al. Prospective, randomized, double-blind assessment of topical bakuchiol and retinol for facial photoageing. Br J Dermatol 2019; 180(2): 289296.

Diepgen T.L., Elsner P., Schliemann S., Fartasch M., Kollner A., Skudlik C., John S.M., Worm M. Guideline on the management of hand eczema ICD-10 Code: L20. L23. L24. L25. L30. J Dtsch Dermatol Ges 2009; 7(Suppl 3): S1–S16.

Diffey B. Sunscreen claims, risk management and consumer confidence. Int J Cosmet Sci 2020; 42(1): 1–4.

Draelos Z.D, Pugliese P.T. Physiology of the skin. 3rd ed. Allured Books, 2011.

Draelos Z.D. Topical agents used in association with cosmetic surgery. Semin Cutan Med Surg 1999; 18(2): 112–118.

Edmonds-Wilson S.L., Nurinova N.I., Zapka C.A., Fierer N., Wilson M. Review of human hand microbiome research. J Dermatol Sci 2015; 80(1): 3–12.

Fowler J.F., Eichenfield L.F., Elias P.M., et al. The chemistry of skin cleansers: an overview for clinicians. Semin Cutan Med Surg 2013; 32(2 Suppl 2): S25–S27.

Gfatter R., Hackl P., Braun F. Effects of soaps and detergents on skin surface pH, stratum corneum hydration and fat content in infants. Dermatology 1997; 195(3): 258–262.

Golden S., Shaw T. Hand dermatitis: review of clinical features and treatment options. Semin Cutan Med Surg 2013; 32(3): 147–157.

Grimes P.E. Jessner's Solution. In: Tosti A., Grimes P.E., De Padova M.P., eds. Color Atlas of Chemical Peels. Berlin, Heidelberg: Springer; 2006.

Grove G.L., Kligman A.M. Corenocyte size as an indirect measure of epidermal proliferative activity. In: Marks R, Plewig G, eds. Stratum corneum. Berlin: Springer Verlag, 1983: 191–195.

Guéniche A., Bastien P., Ovigne J.M., et al. Bifidobacterium longum lysate, a new ingredient for reactive skin. Exp Dermatol 2010; 19(8): e1–e8.

Gunathilake H.M., Sirimana G.M., Schoerer N.Y. The pH of commercially available rinse-off products in Sri Lanka and their effect on skin pH. Ceylon Med J 2007; 52(4): 125–139.

Hernandez E.I., Yutskovskaya Y.A. NEW COSMETOLOGY. Fundamentals of Modern Cosmetology. 2nd ed. Moscow: Cosmetics & Medicine, 2019.

Hikima R., Igarashi S., Ikeda N., et al. Development of lip treatment on the basis of desquamation mechanism. IFSCC Mag 2004; 7: 3–10.

Hines J., Wilkinson S.M., John S.M., Diepgen T.L., English J., Rustemeyer T., Wassilew S., Kezic S., Maibach H.I. The three moments of skin cream application: an evidence-based proposal for use of skin creams in the prevention of irritant contact dermatitis in the workplace. J Eur Acad Dermatol Venereol 2017; 31(1): 53–64.

Huang C., Ma W., Stack S. The hygienic efficacy of different hand-drying methods: a review of the evidence. Mayo Clinic Proceedings 2012; 87(8): 791–798.

Hung S.J., Tang S.C., Liao P.Y., et al. Photoprotective Potential of Glycolic Acid by Reducing NLRC4 and AIM2 Inflammasome Complex Proteins in UVB Radiation-Induced Normal Human Epidermal Keratinocytes and Mice. DNA Cell Biol 2017; 36(2): 177–187.

Ibler K.S., Jemec G.B., Diepgen T.L., Gluud C., Lindschou Hansen J., Winkel P., Thomsen S.F., Agner T. Skin care education and individual counselling versus treatment as usual in healthcare workers with hand eczema: randomised clinical trial. BMJ 2012; 345: e7822.

Imokawa G. A possible mechanism underlying the ceramide deficiency in atopic dermatitis: expression of a deacylase enzyme that cleaves the N-acyl linkage of sphingomyelin and glucosylceramide. J. Dermatol Sci 2009; 55(1): 1–9.

Ishikawa J., Shimotoyodome Y., Ito S., et al. Variations in the ceramide profile in different seasons and regions of the body contribute to stratum corneum functions. Arch Dermatol Res 2013; 305(2): 151–162.

Jaffary F., Faghihi G., Saraeian S., Hosseini S.M. Comparison the effectiveness of pyruvic acid 50% and salicylic acid 30% in the treatment of acne. J Res Med Sci 2016; 21: 31.

Janney M.S., Subramaniyan R., Dabas R., et al. A Randomized Controlled Study Comparing the Efficacy of Topical 5% Tranexamic Acid Solution versus 3% Hydroquinone Cream in Melasma. J Cutan Aesthet Surg 2019; 12(1): 63–67.

Khalil S., Bardawil T., Stephan C., et al. Retinoids: a journey from the molecular structures and mechanisms of action to clinical uses in dermatology and adverse effects. J Dermatolog Treat 2017; 28(8): 684–696.

Kim M.S., Bang S.H., Kim J.H., et al. Tranexamic Acid Diminishes Laser-Induced Melanogenesis. Ann Dermatol 2015; 27(3): 250–256.

Kiousi D.E., Karapetsas A., Karolidou K., et al. Probiotics in Extraintestinal Diseases: Current Trends and New Directions. Nutrients 2019; 11(4): 788.

Kleesz P., Darlenski R., Fluhr J.W. Full-body skin mapping for six biophysical parameters: baseline values at 16 anatomical sites in 125 human subjects. Skin Pharmacol Physiol 2012; 25(1): 25–33.

Kobayashi H., Tagami H. Distinct locational differences observable in biophysical functions of the facial skin: with special emphasis on the poor functional properties of the stratum corneum of the perioral region. Int J Cosmetic Sci 2004; 26: 91–101.

Krężel W., Rühl R., de Lera A.R. Alternative retinoid X receptor (RXR) ligands. Mol Cell Endocrinol 2019; 491: 110436.

Kuehl B.L., Fyfe K.S., Shear N.H. Cutaneous cleansers. Skin Therapy Lett 2003; 8(3): 1–4.

Larson E. Skin hygiene and infection prevention: more of the same or different approaches? Clin Infect Dis 1999; 29: 1287–1294.

Lee B., Heo J., Hong S., et al. DL-Malic acid as a component of α-hydroxy acids: effect on 2,4-dinitrochlorobenzene-induced inflammation in atopic dermatitis-like skin lesions in vitro and in vivo. Immunopharmacol Immunotoxicol 2019; 41(6): 614–621.

Makino E.T., Mehta R.C., Banga A., et al. Evaluation of a hydroquinone-free skin brightening product using in-vitro inhibition of melanogenesis and clinical reduction of ultraviolet-induced hyperpigmentation. J Drugs Dermatol 2013; 12(3): s16–s20.

Miri A., Akbarpour Birjandi S., Sarani M. Survey of cytotoxic and UV protection effects of biosynthesized cerium oxide nanoparticles. J Biochem Mol Toxicol 2020; 34(6): e22475.

Misery L., Ständer S., Szepietowski J.C., et al. Definition of sensitive skin: an expert position paper from the special interest group on sensitive skin of the international forum for the Study of Itch. Acta Derm Venereol 2017; 97(1): 4–6.

Moldovan M., Nanu A. Influence of cleansing product type on several skin parameters after single use. Farmacia 2010; 58(1): 29–37.

Mollerup A., Veien N.K., Johansen J.D. Chronic hand eczema — self-management and prognosis: a study protocol for a randomised clinical trial. BMC Dermatol 2012; 12: 6.

Mottin V.H.M., Suyenaga E.S. An approach on the potential use of probiotics in the treatment of skin conditions: acne and atopic dermatitis. Int J Dermatol 2018; 57(12): 1425–1432.

Muizzuddin N., Maher W., Sullivan M., et al. Physiological effect of a probiotic on skin. J Cosmet Sci 2012; 63(6): 385–395.

Mutters R., Warnes S.L. The method used to dry washed hands affects the number and type of transient and residential bacteria remaining on the skin. J Hosp Infect 2019; 101(4): 408–413.

Na J.I., Shin J.W., Choi H.R., et al. Resveratrol as a Multifunctional Topical Hypopigmenting Agent. Int J Mol Sci 2019; 20(4): 956.

Nikalji N., Godse K., Sakhiya J., et al. Complications of medium depth and deep chemical peels. J Cutan Aesthet Surg 2012; 5(4): 254–260.

Pai V.V., Bhandari P., Shukla P. Topical peptides as cosmeceuticals. Indian J Dermatol Venereol Leprol 2017; 83(1): 9–18.

Park H.J., Cho J.H., Hong S.H., et al. Whitening and anti-wrinkle activities of ferulic acid isolated from Tetragonia tetragonioides in B16F10 melanoma and CCD-986sk fibroblast cells. J Nat Med 2018; 72(1): 127–135.

Park J.B., Lee S.H., Kim K.J., Lee G.Y., Yang J.M., Kim do W., Lee S.J., Lee C.H., Park E.J., Kim K.H., et al. clinical features and awareness of hand eczema in Korea. Ann Dermatol 2016; 28(3): 335–343.

Parrado C., Mercado-Saenz S., Perez-Davo A., et al. Environmental Stressors on Skin Aging. Mechanistic Insights. Front Pharmacol 2019; 10: 759.

Patrick D., Findon G., Miller T. Residual moisture determines the level of touch-contact-associated bacterial transfer following hand washing. Epidemiol Infect 1997; 119(3): 319–325.

Peres D.D., Sarruf F.D., de Oliveira C.A., et al. Ferulic acid photoprotective properties in association with UV filters: multifunctional sunscreen with improved SPF and UVA-PF. J Photochem Photobiol B 2018; 185: 46–49.

Pickart L. The human tripeptide GHK and tissue remodeling. J Biomater Sci Polym Ed 2008; 19(8): 969–988.

Pratchyapruit W., Kikuchi K., Gritiyarangasan P., Aiba S., Tagami H. Functional analyses of the eyelid skin constituting the most soft and smooth area on the face: contribution of its remarkably large superficial corneocytes to effective water-holding capacity of the stratum corneum. Skin Res Technol 2007; 13(2): 169–175.

Riahi R.R., Bush A.E., Cohen P.R. Topical Retinoids: Therapeutic Mechanisms in the Treatment of Photodamaged Skin. Am J Clin Dermatol 2016; 17(3): 265–276.

Salam A., Dadzie O.E., Galadari H. Chemical peeling in ethnic skin: an update. Br J Dermatol 2013; 169(Suppl 3): 82–90.

Sarkar R., Bansal S., Garg V.K. Chemical peels for melasma in dark-skinned patients. J Cutan Aesthet Surg 2012; 5(4): 247–253.

Schagen S.K. Topical Peptide Treatments with Effective Anti-Aging Results. Cosmetics 2017: 4(2); 16.

Schwensen J.F., Friis U.F., Menné T., Johansen J.D. One thousand cases of severe occupational contact dermatitis. Contact Dermatitis 2013; 68(5): 259–268.

Sharad J. Glycolic acid peel therapy — a current review. Clin Cosmet Invest Dermatol 2013; 6: 281–288.

Shimotoyodome Y., Tsujimura H., Ishikawa J., et al. Variations of ceramide profile in different regions of the body of Japanese females. J Jap Cosmet Sci Soc 2014; 38(1): 3–8.

Shriner D.L., Maibach H.I. Regional variation of nonimmunologic contact urticaria. Functional map of the human face. Skin Pharmacol Appl 1996; 9: 312–321.

Smith S. A review of hand washing techniques in primary care and community settings. J Clin Nurs 2009; 18(6): 786–790.

Smith W.P., Bishop M., Gillis G., Maibach H. Topical proteolytic enzymes affect epidermal and dermal properties. Int J Cosmet Sci 2007; 29(1): 15–21.

Soltanipoor M., Kezic S., Sluiter J. K., Rustemeyer T. The effectiveness of a skin care program for the prevention of contact dermatitis in health careworkers (the Healthy Hands Project): study protocol for a cluster randomized controlled trial. Trials 2017; 18(1): 92.

Sondenheimer K., Krutmann J. Novel means for photoprotection. Front Med (Lausanne) 2018; 5: 162.

Stahl W., Sies H. β-Carotene and other carotenoids in protection from sunlight. Am J Clin Nutr 2012; 96(5): 1179–1184.

Surber C., Abels C., Maibach H. pH of the Skin: Issues and Challenges. Current Problems in Dermatology. Basel: Karger; 2018. vol. 54. p. 132–142.

Tamburic S. Changing the skin surface pH: development of the skin surface pH after washing with soaps and handwash liquids. Parfumerie & Kosmetik 1999; 80: 44–46.

Tamura E., Ishikawa J., Yasuda Y., Yamamoto T. The efficacy of synthetic pseudo-ceramide for dry and rough lips. Int J Cosmet Sci 2020 Nov 30.

Tamura E., Yasumori H., Yamamoto T. The efficacy of a highly occlusive formulation for dry lips. Int J Cosmet Sci 2020; 42(1): 46–52.

Tang S.-C., Yang J.-H. Dual Effects of Alpha-Hydroxy Acids on the Skin. Molecules 2018; 23(4): 863.

Tasić-Kostov M., Lukić M., Savić S. A 10% Lactobionic acid-containing moisturizer reduces skin surface pH without irritation-An in vivo/in vitro study. J Cosmet Dermatol 2019; 18(6): 1705–1710.

Tay S.S., Roediger B., Tong P.L., et al. The Skin-Resident Immune Network. Curr Dermatol Rep 2013; 3(1): 13-22.

Todd E.C.D., Michaels B.S., Smith D., Greig J.D., Bartleson C.A. Outbreaks where food workers have been implicated in the spread of foodborne disease, part 9: washing and drying of hands to reduce microbial contamination. J Food Prot 2010; 73(10): 1937–1955.

TRGS 401 Gefährdung durch hautkontakt — ermittlung, beurteilung, Maßnahmen. 2008. www.baua.de/nn_54598/en/Topics-from-A-to-Z/Hazardous-Substances/TRGS/pdf/TRGS-401.pdf.

van der Kolk T., van der Wall H.E.C., Balmforth C., et al. A systematic literature review of the human skin microbiome as biomarker for dermatological drug development. Br J Clin Pharmacol 2018; 84(10): 2178–2193.

Van Gils R.F., van der Valk P.G., Bruynzeel D., Coenraads P.J., Boot C.R., van Mechelen W., Anema J.R. Integrated, multidisciplinary care for hand eczema: design of a randomized controlled trial and cost-effectiveness study. BMC Public Health 2009; 9: 438.

Vandegrift R., Bateman A.C., Siemens K.N., Nguyen M., Wilson H.E., Green J.L., Van Den Wymelenberg K.G., Hickey R.J. Cleanliness in context: reconciling hygiene with a modern microbial perspective. Microbiome 2017; 5(1): 76.

Veien N.K., Hattel T., Laurberg G. Hand eczema: causes, course, and prognosis I. Contact Dermatitis 2008; 58(6): 330–334.

Walters R.M., Mao G., Gunn E.T., Hornby S. Cleansing formulations that respect skin barrier integrity. Dermatol Res Pract 2012; 2012: 495917.

WHO encourages patient participation for hand hygiene in health care. News Release 2013. www.who.int/mediacentre/news/releases/2013/hand_hygiene_20130503/en.

Yevglevskis M., Bowskill C.R., Chan C.C., et al. A study on the chiral inversion of mandelic acid in humans. Org Biomol Chem 2014; 12(34): 6737–6744.

Yokota T., Matsumoto M., Sakamaki T. Classification of sensitive skin and development of treatment system appropriate for each group. IFSCC Magazine 2003; 6: 303–307.

Zapka C., Leff J., Henley J., Tittl J., De Nardo E., Butler M., et al. Comparison of standard culture-based method to culture-independent method for evaluation of hygiene effects on the hand microbiome. MBio 2017; 8(2).

Zdrada J., Odrzywołek W., Deda A., et al. A split-face comparative study to evaluate the efficacy of 50% pyruvic acid against a mixture of glycolic and salicylic acids in the treatment of acne vulgaris. J Cosmet Dermatol 2020; 19(9): 2352–2358.

Zhou H., Zhao J., Li A., Reetz M.T. Chemical and Biocatalytic Routes to Arbutin. Molecules 2019; 24(18): 3303.

Zlotogorski A. Distribution of the skin pH on the forehead and cheek of adult. Arch Dermatol Res 1987; 279: 398–401.

Zubair S., Mujtaba G. Comparison of efficacy of topical 2% liquiritin, topical 4% liquiritin and topical 4% hydroquinone in the management of melasma. J Pakistan Assoc Dermatologist 2009; 19: 158–163.

www.ingramcontent.com/pod-product-compliance
Lightning Source LLC
Chambersburg PA
CBHW052019030426
42335CB00026B/3204